FOOD FREEDOM

A Faith-Based, Holistic Approach to Shift You from Defeat to Victory Over Emotional Eating

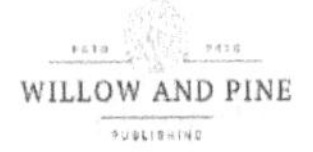

LINDSAY WENDLAND

Food Freedom: A Faith-Based, Holistic Approach to Shift You from Defeat to Victory Over Emotional Eating

Published by Willow and Pine

Somerset, WI 54025

ISBN: 978-0-578-39663-7

Cover Art: "The Storm" by Monique Green

First Printing 2021

DEDICATION

For my daughters, Aubrey, Brenna, and Grace: you make me brave and bold.

For the Titus 2 women who have been my teachers: it was the freedom in Christ I saw in you that let me know it was possible.

Table of Contents

FOOD FREEDOM

IT'S NOT SUPPOSED TO BE THIS WAY WITH FOOD

I Know What it is to be Imprisoned and I Know What it is to be Free

FOR 36 YEARS, I was entangled in an out-of-order relationship with food. I was imprisoned in my thoughts and emotions, held captive to shame and self-hate within my body.

I believed I would never be free from the bondage of food, the vicious cycle of restriction, and the aftermath of when I fully lost control. Cupboards, drive-throughs, pantries, and refrigerators were where I ran for safety. They were my gods and sources of comfort.

As a preschooler, I emptied the full cookie jar at Grandma's house in a matter of one hour. I hid in closets and bathrooms, eating cookie after cookie, not even tasting them. I lived with an overwhelming feeling of emptiness and pain. My little hands reached for anything they could find, in the hopes of filling a void.

As I got older, my weekend cycles turned into daily after-school binges. I opened the front door to an empty house and opened cupboard doors and packages like my life depended upon it. I stuffed down potato chips, cookies, sandwiches, and cereal until time ran out; I had to hide what I consumed. After my food frenzy, I sat at the table with my parents for dinner, pretending I had not just consumed thousands of calories.

I collapsed into bed each night, holding my stomach, so full, and on the cusp of bursting. I prayed to God for help and vowed to myself, and Him, that I would never eat that way again.

Each morning I greeted the day with the hope that I could end it without losing control. But every night I curled over my over-stuffed stomach, praying, and vowing again.

My body size, and weight, climbed every year in school. I wasn't just the fat kid, I was morbidly obese and the butt of every joke. But I couldn't stop eating, no matter how hard I tried.

By the age of nineteen, I was well over three hundred pounds and had almost given over to the belief that I would always struggle with food and be overweight. I believed I had no power to stop it. I believed food ruled my life.

But underneath layers of hiding, and years of coping was a still, small Voice that whispered, "You were made for more than this," and "It's not supposed to be this way."

By twenty-five I was lost, homeless, divorced and living the life of an addict. Not only was I still using food, but dove headfirst into alcohol, drugs, and men. I used whatever I could find to scratch the itch and quell the emptiness deep inside of me.

I believed the lie that I would never be free while feeling the nudge and hearing the whisper that freedom could also be mine. I walked tightropes, balancing between a taught faith in God that I didn't yet understand and continuing to take matters into my own hands. I believed no one was coming for me, no one was going to save me, and I was all alone in my mess. But it wasn't supposed to be that way, and still isn't.

I finally found what I was looking for all along: the answer to my inner strife, the quell to my traumatized and fractured heart. But it wasn't a thing I found, but Someone standing with me at the bottom of my pit: Christ.

He was there all along, in the depth of my despair, holding a candle and ushering out the darkness. It was finally time for me to see Him, and recognize Jesus as a Friend, not a foe. I was ready to be rescued and saved from myself, acknowledging that Someone did come for me and had a plan all along.

~

It's been fifteen years since I met Jesus in my prison, and He offered me a key. These years have been filled with so much goodness and change, along with so much heartache and pain. I had to learn that my food issues weren't keeping God and His love from me, but I was the one allowing my failures and issues to keep me from God. He beckons us to bring all these things to the table, allowing Him to take them on and hash them out. He reminds us that they are already dealt with and dead and in the grave.

It's humans that put God in a box to try to explain Him, understand Him, and even control Him. But God is just asking us to walk with Him, commune with Him, be in a relationship with Him, and love Him back.

To know the voice of God we must read His Word and learn His character. We must surrender ourselves repeatedly, to His will and His ways.

We want freedom so badly, yet we are often unwilling to do the one thing we must do for freedom: let go of ourselves and trust that He will care for us completely. Freedom is a gift for us to believe, receive, and accept as ours. But total food freedom can only be found in Christ. This is the way it's supposed to be because you and I were made for more than just conforming to the way the world does things and looking like everyone else.

We will still walk tensions and tightropes, understanding that we are to steward and surrender these lives, all the while knowing He has already given us everything we need.

My freedom from food was thirty-six years in the making, but I am grateful that it didn't come any sooner. I had to be ready to do the work to get free and stay free.

In all transparency, I used food to stuff and numb out extreme brokenness and pain. My brain was trying to keep me safe and comfortable from an abounding source of discomfort. As a child, I wasn't supposed to have been faced with what I was faced with. I wasn't supposed to feel, hear, or see the things that I did. Trauma caused a chasm within my soul and a felt brokenness that I carried within my body.

My disordered eating was a response to trauma, and until I was ready to fully face the pain that I carried, I was not ready to break free. But inch by inch and step by step, I was led to learn how to stand up for myself, stand on my own two feet and walk forward. I came to a point where I hated my sin so much, and I hated what it taught me.

Our bodies hold our stories, whether we know our story, or not.

Our souls keep count and recollect what has transpired, even if we consciously have no idea.

At the end of the day, it's not about a diet plan, it's not about weight loss, it's about healing those broken places within your heart so that you can and will be free from them. Healing needs to come to our emotions and our ways of thinking so that we may steward this body well and the life that God has given us to fulfill. It looks like a lot of forgiveness, feeling the pain of the past so that future triggers won't be "pushed down." It looks like seeing things from a different perspective and with a new lens on yourself and your life. It looks like taking off your old way of thinking, and coming out of agreement with thought patterns that only bring death. Healing looks like accepting God's Word and Will for your life, and then running whole-heartedly with them, with Him by your side.

Every failed diet, weight loss attempt, and painful Day One had to come to pass so that I could learn how to be planted on the foundation of Truth.

I had to go back into my life, with a lit path from God, face my demons, and boldly claim "No more!" I had to come to the end of myself, hate my sin, and come out of the agreement that I needed to continue feeding my feelings and numbing my pain.

"The answer to your pain is in your pain." – Alisa Keeton, Founder of Revelation Wellness.

Let's gather up all the places life has taken us, shake the dust from our feet, and realize that it has all been for such a time as this. All the attempts, wins, losses, money spent, and tears cried over a sleeve of cookies are back in yesterday. They do not define you, nor do they get a say in who you are today or tomorrow.

There are several separations and reframes I want to address as we get started:

1) Healing emotional eating and losing weight are two separate things—they can be done simultaneously but focusing on healing FIRST will lead to better results down the road (less yo-yoing).

2) Depending on your current state of emotional/binge eating, success will look different. Since I was a daily binger, going one week was my first big victory.

3) Celebrate success in new ways. Gone are the days when sticking to your diet for x number of days then allowing yourself to binge is something you will do. You are not a dog; do not reward good behavior with food. You were made for more. Celebrate differently.

4) Perfectionism is from the pit of hell. It is rooted in pride

and will get you a one-way ticket to frustration and overwhelm. We don't do that here.

5) Understand that healing is messy and often things get worse before they get better. During my window of healing intense emotions, I had one of the biggest binges of my life. It was the first and only time in thirty-six years of emotional eating that I threw up and was concerned my stomach would burst.

6) The enemy doesn't want you free. He will do anything in his power to knock you off track, get you distracted, and circle the drain to your demise.

Remember, the enemy is the enemy. You, your body, your spouse, children, parents, work, or neighbors are not the enemy. Food is not your enemy, and not even your emotions are the enemy. The enemy is the enemy, and we will fight as such.

7) Your brain will want you to remember all the diets and ways of doing things before. When things get tough (I call it getting jiggy) it may seem easier to quit pressing in and pushing on in the way we do things here. But as Pastor Steven Furtick said in his sermon about the Israelites marching around Jericho seven times, "Don't stop on six."

Your breakthrough may be just around the corner from you, so continue to march on.

TAKE BACK YOUR TERRITORY

Stop Allowing Life to Happen Around You and To You

YEARS AGO, THE LORD prompted me to start coaching and writing based on an idea that we need to "take back our territory." I sought the Lord, asking "What is this territory? How did it get stolen? And why must it be taken back?" I used to think the territory was something outside of myself, something I was to go out and take or go after. But the more I found the Lord, and He healed parts of me and my life, I learned that **I am the territory that must be taken back.** The territories we need to take back are within ourselves and our lives. And we begin with learning to steward (take responsibility) for ourselves spiritually, mentally, emotionally, and physically.

Being believers, and temples of the Holy Spirit, we have been given everything we need for life and godliness (2 Peter 1:3). But somewhere along the way, this belief was stolen.

Whether you grew up in a Christian home or not.

Whether you knew Jesus when you sucked your thumb or are just getting to know Him now.

Being a believer is so much more than just showing up to a worship service on Sunday and checking the "church box" for the week.

As believers, we are co-creators and co-heirs with Christ. Not only do we get the deposit of the Holy Spirit within us, but everything that is Christ's in the Kingdom of God is ours too.

The more territory we take back and surrender to the Lord, the more of His Kingdom we get to experience in our lives. Jesus often said, "The Kingdom of Heaven is upon you."

His kingdom is here on earth, up for grabs, and here for the taking.

Nothing pleases the Father more than His kids fully believing in His Son, Jesus, and running with every inspired word that was written and spoken to us by His Holy Spirit.

What if we truly "threw off the weight and the sin that so easily entangles us and run with endurance, this race set before us, fixing our eyes on Jesus, the Author and Perfector of our faith." (Hebrews 12:1)

What if the tension and ferocity you feel within you, or what comes against the bondage you are dealing with in life, is the

Holy Spirit at work within you, begging you to come up higher? To take on His perspective is to see that your food issue is already dead and buried in the grave. The cycle, pattern, and habit have already been taken care of. And you have been declared free, according to His plan, purpose, and goodness.

The Holy Spirit is zealously cheering for you to understand that everything you are struggling with is already under your feet because you are in Christ.

Say this declaration:

"Emotional and binge eating are under my feet. They are dead in the grave. They don't get to speak over me, control me, define me, or have any say in my choices moving forward. Jesus came, died, and was resurrected for my freedom, and I will walk in the fullness of that freedom. In Jesus' name, Amen."

Let's take back your territory from food today, and for the rest of your life.

I categorize our territories (what we are responsible to steward and surrender back to the Lord) in four areas:

1) Spiritual

2) Emotional

3) Mental

4) Physical

Each territory is built upon the same four pillars:

1) Word of God

2) Prayer

3) Intimacy with our Heavenly Father

4) Identity rooted in Christ

When we go after freedom, healing, and making life-long changes, we must "take on" each one of these areas. I don't know about you, but I have a love/hate relationship with confrontation. It's uncomfortable but necessary to continue to move forward throughout life.

Most of the work you will do in *Food Freedom* will be done in a spirit of confrontation. You will:

Confront your habits

Emotional eating has nothing to do with food and has everything to do with your emotions and learned habits.

Confront counterfeit teachings rooted in a fear-based diet-culture

The problem and the reason you have been kept in this cycle is you have been using a physical thing to fix an emotional issue. Diet culture, and people who don't understand emotional eating, will feed you the tall tale that more disciplined eating is the fix for your emotional eating.

Confront lies you've been believing about yourself.

I don't know about you, but I've experienced tons of shame, guilt and condemnation from following rules and diets that never fixed my emotional eating. There is no shame in the struggle, because this isn't about willpower, but giving permission and honor to your emotions and separating from using food.

SPIRITUAL TERRITORY

Come Back to Your Original Design as Beloved and Whole.

I equate spiritual territory with our relationship to God, His Son, and the Holy Spirit.

Religion likes to teach us rules to follow and laws to abide by. It seems easier to categorize and classify ourselves according to pass or fail. Rules and religion also make it easier for us to make up our minds about God and His goodness.

Our spiritual territory begins in our relationship with God and how we relate to Him. We can learn that our earthly father did not 100% reflect our Heavenly Father, maybe not even 1%. As we grow, we can discern the differences and find our misgivings about God may have been projected from a place of pain, or ideals that simply were not characteristics of Him at all, but something that man thought up to understand or justify his actions.

How we relate to God is everything, and how He relates to us is even greater still.

*"Now they have come to know that
everything which You have given Me is
from You; for the words which You gave
Me I have given to them; and they
received them and truly understood that
I came forth from You, and they believed
that You sent Me. I ask on their behalf; I
do not ask on behalf of the world, but on
the behalf of those whom You have given
Me, because they are Yours; all things
that are Mine are Yours, and Yours are
Mine; and I have been glorified in them. I
am no longer going to be in the world;
and yet they themselves are in the world,
and I am coming to You. Holy Father,
keep them in Your name, the name which
You have given Me, so that they may be
one just as We are."*

John 17:7-11

We can take back our territory from sin and what was stolen and live our "new creation" lives with joy unending and unyielding. We can live in God's Kingdom while being on earth, a life of freedom and fruit of what Jesus did for us on the Cross.

What starts with salvation prayer can lead to a beautiful and brilliant relationship with your Creator. He is the One who knows you best and loves you most. Not only do we get to know Him, but we also get to be used by Him, for His kingdom and glory. We get to have a relationship with Almighty God, unveiled because of Christ.

He is not just God on the mountaintop, He is God on the bathroom floor. He is God that kneels and stoops low to breathe life into us. He is God that bankrupted heaven to come to be with us and save us.

EMOTIONAL TERRITORY

Give Yourself Permission to Feel and Honor your Emotions with Grace and Truth.

On every coaching call, I ask the same question:

"How are you taking care of yourself emotionally?"

I ask this question after my client tells me all the choices they have been making with food and how they have been moving their bodies. They know the timing of their meals, calorie intake, and how many sweat sessions they had for the week. The conversation often morphs into them revealing they found themselves out of control when they stumbled upon their child's Halloween candy bag or the donut box in the break room at work.

Some of my clients have full-on binges like I used to, but most of them are just overeating and not able to maintain self-control around certain foods and at certain times.

I ask them about the care of their emotions, and they are often stumped, unable to provide an answer. You may have learned early on in life that your emotions are not important or are invalid. You may have been told that you are too sensitive or too much. Maybe someone else's emotional state became more important than yours.

As women, we are taught not to "be too emotional" if we are to ever get ahead in the world. But in doing so, we are often stripped of what makes us who we are and how we feel about things. Giving yourself and those around you permission to fully feel their feelings validates more than just their emotions. This empathetic act also acknowledges the person and their humanity.

Taking back your emotional territory gives honor to who you are and how you feel while maintaining the truth and the essence of who you truly are.

You have permission to fully feel and honor your emotions, rather than negating and stuffing them, thereby falling into self-harm.

> *"Keep your heart with all vigilance, for*
> *from it flow the springs of life."*
>
> *Proverbs 4:23*

MENTAL TERRITORY

The Battlefield for Your Freedom Begins and Ends in Your Mind.

I could line this entire book with quotes and scripture about mental territory and it still wouldn't exhaustively convey how important your thoughts are.

Everything you say, do, and feel begins with a single thought.

One of the biggest lies going around is that you cannot control your thoughts. But I say if you have control over one thing, and one thing only, it is your thoughts.

Your thoughts are what make you human, not being led by primal sub-conscious drivers.

Have you ever thought about what you are thinking about? Your brain is always telling a story. There is always a narrative playing, speaking, and telling. As our subconscious began recording and storing files of information, all the way back to the 3rd trimester in the womb, our brains began to tell us a story.

Our mind forms perceptions about ourselves and the world around us.

Pain is registered and stored. Trauma is recorded and held.

Words spoken are taken note of. And whether our emotional, mental, and physical needs were met, or not, that was recorded and organized too. Our brains protect us and keep us surviving no matter what. And until we learn differently, or until we see a different way offered to us, we will generally take whatever information about ourselves and the world we can get.

Your mental territory is much more than what you think. We will create a foundational work in this book and program, but please understand my heart when I say your mental health is the most important thing you can take care of, only second to spiritual health.

> *"As a man thinks in his heart, so is he."*
>
> *Proverbs 23:7*

PHYSICAL TERRITORY

Break Up with Old Agreements About Your Body

What used to be a place of contention for me is now a space of compassion.

But growing from the mindset that I needed to bully myself into a smaller body was a journey of missteps, redirects, and full of frustration.

I had to remove the idea that being at war with myself, and my body, was the way to health and wholeness. The years I spent chastising myself, restricting food to the point of starvation, and running hundreds of miles to burn off bad choices were rooted in fear and misunderstanding.

In taking back the territory of my body, I had to learn how to become my friend. I had to start speaking to myself and my body as a true friend would speak to me. A true friend would be honest and not hide from showing me my blind spots but would do so lovingly and kindly. A true friend would speak and act with kindness, but also boldness to knock the doughnut out of my hand when I was in self-pity mode. Compassion had to move into my mindset and thinking when it came to my body. But compassion doesn't grab a fork and eat the cake with you. True compassion, like Jesus, acknowledges the pain and emotions but also calls you to a standard of thinking and living that is above your circumstance.

We are to be advocates for our bodies, not enemies.

We are not to bow to disease, but to do what we can to prevent it. Our days can be filled with advancing the kingdom of God and glorifying His name, not focused solely on the limitations of our physicality.

Taking back the territory of your body and physical health is so much more than your weight on the scale or waistline. It is about stewarding your body, the temple of the Holy Spirit, so that you may run with endurance the race set before you, able to show up to the call of God every single day and in every circumstance.

The enemy wants nothing more than for you to be focused on your body and whatever eating habits you have. If you are constantly looking down, you are not looking into the face of your Creator. God is calling you into a place of rest and wholeness, but also into a space of boldness and ferocity to move His kingdom forward.

> *"The enemy comes only to kill,*
> *steal, and destroy, but I have come*
> *to bring you life and life*
> *abundant."*
>
> *John 10:10*

1

SEPARATE HUNGER

Let's Stop Filling Up on What Does Not Satisfy

I STOOD IN FRONT OF OPEN refrigerator doors, not hungry, but looking for something to quell a nagging hunger within me. I've driven through restaurants with bags of food handed to me from a sliding glass window, with the only intention of stuffing whatever feeling I was unwilling to feel at the time. I've spent hours thinking about the perfect binge meal: McDonald's fries, a chicken sandwich from Burger King, and dessert from DQ. Once the last bite was consumed, I was still unsatisfied, feeling even more empty inside than before I began.

It is something to feel so empty and bottomless, while on the verge of exploding from an over-stuffed stomach and strained esophagus.

The hopelessness of emotional eating kept me company for almost four decades.

There was a war within me, and the battle being fought was whether I believed I had a choice in the matter.

Bondage and addiction make you believe that you must keep choosing them, that there is no other way.

The needle calls to the junkie.

The bottle sings its sad song to the alcoholic.

The sleeve of cookies whispers softly, yet firmly, to the eater.

The undercurrent of our vice's voice tells us that we simply cannot live without them, let alone get through the next ten minutes without using them.

These self-inflicted masters want you to believe that you have no option but to follow them into oblivion. Heeding their calls, you come running.

This is addiction at its finest: loving and hating the idol we created all at once.

But I am here to let you in on what I found out when I looked further at my taskmaster. The legs on which they stand are unfounded and quite the masquerade. They are nothing but lip service, covering up our primal need and desire to feel safe and well taken care of.

These needs were set into motion at our creation; we were made this way. You and I have a God-sized hole within our hearts that can only be filled with God Himself. The more we go after attempting to fill this void with worldly things, the larger and stronger it becomes.

But I believe you are at a place today where you have realized the way you have been doing things no longer serves you. You have come to the end of the ride; you want off the carousel and to leave this amusement park completely. Gone are the days where rollercoasters are fun, and maybe sitting in the sun with a big cup of peace feels like Heaven on Earth.

> *"The Kingdom of God is not what*
> *you eat or drink, but righteousness,*
> *peace, and joy in the Holy Spirit."*
> *Romans 14:17*

Let's learn how to separate the hunger within us so that we can be filled in an everlasting way.

CREATED TO CRAVE

You Were Created to Crave Relationship with God

We were created in the likeness and the Image of God. He is relational, and so are we. Everything God does is in relationship to Himself and His character.

God loves because He is love and all the characteristics that go with love: patience, kindness, not boasting, not arrogant, not dishonoring, not self-seeking, not easily angered, keeping no record of wrongs. Because God is love and love is God, He doesn't delight in evil, but rejoices with the truth, always protecting, trusting, hoping, and persevering (see 1 Corinthians 13).

Because of the fall of man, our ability to relate to God and even relate to the way He loves us is fractured. We project our perceptions upon Him and ourselves in relation to Him. But we have His Word and His Holy Spirit to reveal God's true nature and heart.

God longs to be with us, so much so that He created a rescue plan when we chose fruit over following His commandment in the garden. You are I were created to crave the presence of God in our lives, and nothing else will fill that God-sized hole. Not food, money, or a smaller body. Not even the relationships with our spouses or children can fill it.

We are to recognize this truth, come out of hiding behind closed doors, and stop choosing the things of this world. Things that can only offer us a counterfeit and are merely a bent glimpse of what the Kingdom of Heaven is really like. We must go to God to find what we are truly longing for.

Now that we know better, we can do better.

I believe you and I want the same things:

- To be seen, known, and loved right where and as you are.
- To know, no matter what, that you are fully loved and fully forgiven for whatever has transpired in your life.
- To learn and taste this great mercy, grace, and peace that Christ offers us.

- To fully know that your worth is not tied to your waistline, bank account, job prospect, or status.

You and I long to be longed for, and we get that from our Creator, our Father in Heaven because He does too.

To begin, read John 4: 1-38, seek the Lord, and answer the questions:

Father, what has my heart been craving after that can only be found in You?

What have I been filling my life with that will not truly satisfy?

Jesus, where have I picked up habits and longed after something other than You to satisfy my deepest need?

Holy Spirit, what is my heart hungry for? Show me how God already satisfies this with His presence.

- What will you lay down today, and refuse to pick up again because it is empty and will never satisfy?
- How will you commit this action to the Lord and to yourself?

Father God, You know my heart. You know my wanderings and my misgivings. You know where I have picked things up that did not satisfy my desire for You, and I cannot seem to put them down. Help me see how empty they are, help me put them down and keep them down, knowing that what you offer me us so much greater. You have what I need, living water, and you place within me this well of the Holy Spirit that I get to go to whenever I need. Please dig this well deep within me, that it may never run dry. Show me how to steward it, so that others may drink from it, and You.

SPIRITUAL HUNGER

You Were Made to Worship

You and I were made to worship God and God alone.

We can often feel that God turns and walks away from us when we choose something other than Him.

But it is not Him that moves from us, God is stationary and "the same yesterday, today, and forever" (Hebrews 13:8). We become distant, distracted, and chase after things that are in a different kingdom. We grow tired and weary of waiting for answers to prayers. Our lives get too hectic to take a breath or look for hidden corners of respite. Or maybe we are so used to chaos and disarray that the quiet seems scary and way too big.

Your soul was created to worship God and crave being with Him.

When we worship things, making them our gods, like food, we stop craving the presence of God and begin to crave the counterfeit comfort that food provides us.

Using food for comfort, release, pacifying, or numbing are counterfeit and short-lived fixes that will only lead to more need. We pick emptiness to fill the emptiness and are left confused when we come up empty. In the back of our minds, we acknowledge, "I thought that would help, but it just made me feel more alone and now I'm ashamed that I did it."

We create idols out of these things we go to. We turn to worship them, instead of our Creator God.

We have our morning quiet time, read our pretty devotionals, highlight scripture in our Bible. We go to our place of worship on Sunday mornings and Wednesday nights, but what are we doing with that worship the rest of the time? What are we worshiping the other 166 hours?

Is Jesus staying in the leather-bound Bible or are you taking Him with you into your day?

Or have we become so calloused in our thinking, acting, and reaching for other things that we neglect the presence of God altogether?

If we are to be the Church, and a city set on a hill, then we need to get back to worshiping and craving after God, Who craves us. Gone are the days where seeking God's hand in our lives is enough. If we are ever to get free from food and have our lives set on a course that worships Him alone, we must seek His face, His voice, and His presence.

We must seek to delight Him as we delight in Him.

We must hunger and thirst after God and His presence, not just His power.

When we return to our first love, freedom begins to fall into place. Our sensitivity to the Holy Spirit begins to grow. God's conviction comes like an answered prayer, and we get to rise to the occasion of Him calling us higher.

"'For I know the plans that I have for you,' declares the LORD, 'plans for prosperity and not for disaster, to give you a future and a hope. Then you will call upon Me and come and pray to Me, and I will listen to you. And you will seek Me and find Me when you search for Me with all your heart. I will let Myself be found by you,' declares the LORD, 'and I will restore your fortunes and gather you from all the nations and all the places where I have driven you,' declares the LORD, 'and I will bring you back to the place from where I sent you into exile.'"

Jeremiah 29:11-14

"Blessed are those who hunger and thirst after righteousness, for they shall be satisfied."

Matthew 5:6

Please journal and answer these questions:

- When have you been worshiping something other than your heavenly Father, requiring it to fill the God-sized hole within you?
- Where do your thoughts go when you are feeling overwhelmed, anxious, afraid, or lonely? What do your thoughts say about what will "fix" these feelings? Why are these thoughts wrong?
- What is the better choice you can make when you are feeling this way?
- How will you put these better choices into practice today?

---

*Father, where have I been worshiping
something or someone other than you?
Holy Spirit please reveal to me how this
has affected my life. Father, I only want
to worship you. My heart longs for you,
all that is within me craves You and Your
nearness. I don't want to be distracted
anymore; help me not be distant. Please
show me margin in my days for us to be
together. I come out of agreement that I
need something other than your
presence to make me whole. Please
forgive me for when I have chosen the
world over You. Holy Spirit please remind
me, teach me, and grow me up in the
fullness of spiritual discernment so that I
can see what is trying to kill, steal, and
destroy my relationship with God. I want
to walk in the fullness, wholeness, and
wellness of everything that I am offered
in the Kingdom of God, in Christ Jesus.*

EMOTIONAL HUNGER

Emotional Eating is Often Caught and Taught

Spiritual hunger will send us into overdrive picking up identities we aren't supposed to be carrying and habits we don't want to fall victim to. If we aren't filling ourselves spiritually first, the rest of our efforts will come to no avail. We will worship things not meant to be worshiped and sign up for bondages we didn't want in the first place.

Sometimes inviting Jesus into those places of our heart that need love cures our desires to eat. We can be instantly delivered of those desires and no longer go to food or other things for a "fix."

But most of the time, we get to walk this out, falling on the strength that Christ gives us.

In this fallen world, things are bent and twisted and we can confuse one thing for another.

As children, we looked to our parents and caregivers to lead us in the ways of life. We learned by watching what the people around us did, how they acted and reacted to life.

When you were younger learning how to ride a bicycle, skateboard, or rollerblade, I'm sure you fell a few times. When you skinned your knees, were you scooped up and sat down on the bathroom stool? Were your open wounds anointed with peroxide, anti-bacterial ointment, and a Bugs Bunny adhesive bandage? Were you given ice cream, candy, or a sweet to "make it feel better"?

What did this teach you?

What was celebration like in your home? Did a joyous occasion call for a full spread of home-cooked or store-bought foods?

When someone was upset or stressed in your home, what were their reactions? What did your parents or caregivers go to?

Did you learn that a physical thing can be used to help an emotional issue?

None of these things are bad or wrong, but it can be helpful to recognize what we were taught so we can unlearn them.

Even our society uses commercials and ads to sell us a storyline that things can help us feel better, or not feel at all.

Maybe you are like me: not allowed to display emotions growing up, yet had big feelings and didn't understand emotions, so you turned to a physical thing to stuff and numb.

Maybe you weren't permitted to feel.

Maybe you were told you were too much, not enough, or you should be seen and not heard.

Maybe someone else's emotions were made more important than your own.

And so you had to turn to something to hide your emotions.

Shame likes us to hide and stay hidden, but it's time to remove shame and guilt from emotional eating.

Your brain is wired to keep you safe and comfortable. It will look for answers as it navigates what is going on in the environment around you. Your brain makes up stories, always telling a narrative, posing answers that may not be correct or lack necessary information.

As children, we should have felt loved, nurtured, comforted, and safe. But those felt things are not always a part of our story. Did you reach for something that helped you feel safe, while your environment was not? Did you use food to pacify and survive your situation?

Over the years of doing things this way, using food, a habit was created. Your brain learned and adapted to believe that when you feel an emotion, the answer is to eat.

That's why most of the work you will do to move from frustration to freedom will be done internally. My food freedom journey did not come by fixating on food but came with the understanding that I needed to heal emotionally; food was never going to be the fix. Your emotions are valid and learning how to take care of yourself emotionally, with boundaries and compassion, is a key to food freedom. Let's remove the idea that fixing ourselves physically will fix us emotionally, mentally, or spiritually. Work with yourself, rather than against. Inviting the Holy Spirit into every part of who you are will help that freedom door swing open even faster and wider.

~

We are to honor our emotions, not be governed by them. By honoring your emotions, you will grow in emotional intelligence.

Emotional intelligence is the ability to understand, use, and positively manage your emotions.

Emotionally intelligent people:

- Notice, feel, engage, and steward emotions, but do not surrender to them.
- Surrender to God, not the will of emotions.
- Monitor their emotional state without judgment or self-harm
- Acknowledge feelings with honesty, paying attention with empathy and patience
- Analyze the feeling and give it a name

As believers, we often walk a tightrope between our feelings and God's truth. We do not deny our feelings but put them in the proper place.

When I learned that my unhealthy eating habits were due to my emotions not being managed well, everything changed. I was able to separate my eating habits from my emotions, working on them separately, yet simultaneously.

~

As emotional eaters, we have learned how to manage ourselves and our emotions by stuffing. But to find freedom we must do the opposite: we must heal.

To heal, we must begin to feel.

We heal in the place where emotions drive us to do what we did not want to do but are enslaved to do.

We heal mentally, allowing the Holy Spirit to renew our thoughts about God and ourselves.

We heal in our relationship with food and stop having an emotional relationship with it.

We must also begin to practice acknowledging our feelings, allowing their voice to speak in a safe space, and correctly discerning what to do with them.

These are conscious efforts, in our adult-thinking brain, not in our subconscious (limbic brain) where our emotions are cultivated.

If we are to grow into emotional maturity with the fruit of food freedom, we need a few things first:

1) Safety

2) Permission

3) Information

We need to feel safe to process our emotions—this approach is compassionate and kind. Bringing judgment and shame into the mix negates safety and permission, so they are not invited.

Safety: Where is your space of safety where you can feel, process, and move through your emotions without interruption?

Some ideas:

- Wake early for quiet time and journaling
- In your closet or car
- Prayer walks or nature hikes
- Working in the yard or at a hobby

What ideas or promptings from the Holy Spirit do you have for your safe space?

Permission: Granting yourself permission to feel and move through your emotions is crucial and attached to safety. One of the biggest obstacles with permission is the fear that you will stay stuck in a feeling or thought process. Generally, when you allow yourself to fully feel, ask questions along the way, and don't bring judgment to the table, your process won't be stunted. By inviting the Holy Spirit into your process, He will show you the truth and bring much-needed comfort.

You can compassionately grant yourself permission:

- Permission to fully grieve.
- Permission to fall apart.
- Permission to do what needs to be done so that you don't get stuck in a cycle, but can move through.
- Permission to not act like you have all your stuff together.
- Permission to hope and look for brighter days ahead.

Information: Processing emotions can look different for everyone and sometimes we need an extra hand to get us through. Prayerfully finding a therapist, pastor, counselor, or support group can be very helpful in your healing journey.

Permitting yourself to get help is a huge step. Asking yourself "what do I need?" can be helpful but also overwhelming, because we may not know the answer. Still, allow yourself the crucial time and space to process. When I stopped requiring myself to come up to an expectation of time, I was able to feel safe and permit myself to process through.

When we are willing to see our healing through, our freedom is waiting for us on the other side.

"I will ask the Father, and He will give you another Helper, so that He may be with you forever; the Helper is the Spirit of truth, whom the world cannot receive, because it does not see Him or know Him; but you know Him because He remains with you and will be in you. 'I will not leave you as orphans; I am coming to you.'"

John 14:16-18

What Does Emotional Hunger Feel Like?

As spirit-filled beings in bodies, we have multiple hungers. Our spirit will always be hungering for more God, but our emotions and bodies hunger too.

Often our signals of emotional and physical hunger get twisted, and we end up feeding an emotional issue with physical food.

Emotional hunger:

- Comes on suddenly or abruptly.
- Makes you crave only certain foods
- Creates a binge and you may not be able to sense physical fullness.
- Provokes feelings of shame or guilt about eating after.
- This urge can feel like an insistent "now." I must eat _______ now.

Emotional hunger often feels like something has kicked you out of the driver's seat and is now driving you. You have an urge to eat when you are not physically hungry and might feel out of control or unable to make a healthy choice with food. When I got curious about my emotional hunger, I learned it was rooted in anxiety. I wanted my uncomfortable feelings to be gone in an instant, and I believed the lie that food was my way out.

Food is never the way out.

When you are feeling these sensations, find a safe space, take a big deep breath, and give yourself permission and time to ask a few questions to navigate emotional hunger.

EMOTIONAL HUNGER QUESTIONS

- What am I feeling?
- Why do I feel this way?
- What other times in my life do I feel like this?
- What does this feel like in my body?
- What do I need?
- What do I really want?
- What will I do instead of eating?

"The wisdom of the sensible is to understand his way."

Proverbs 14:8

PHYSICAL HUNGER

What Does it Feel Like to Be Physically Hungry?

When I coached the first group through the *Food Freedom* Intensive, all five of them were shocked at the same thing: they felt true physical hunger for the first time in years, maybe even the first time in their lives.

When I introduced the Hunger Scale, this way of eating prompted my clients to learn how it feels to be truly physically hungry, without fear. They also learned what it means to be physically satisfied and what fullness feels like. It's a beautiful practice getting into your body, truly feeling hunger and satiety, while beginning to restore resistant hormones.

I used to be afraid of feeling hungry. It was because of an orphan heart, poverty, and scarcity mindset. But now I look forward to that groan in my belly; it is an opportunity to turn things over to God and remember His faithfulness to me. As emotional eaters, we may not know what it feels like to be truly physically hungry, or we may be well-acquainted with hunger because we starve ourselves as a "fix" after a binge.

Physical hunger:

- Develops over time, slowly.
- Desires a variety of food groups.
- Cues the sensation of satiety to stop eating.
- Has no negative feelings about eating.

We will begin to recognize some current habits with hunger to start walking this out.

PHYSICAL HUNGER QUESTIONS:

- What am I hungry for?
- What am I feeling in my body?
- What do I need to nourish my body?
- What does my body need to be fed for proper energy?

Practice noticing the difference between emotional and physical hunger by getting curious and investigating what hunger you are truly feeling.

Practice this new awareness before from when you wake in the morning all throughout your day. Become a student of your habits, thoughts, and emotions. Become a student of how hunger feels in your body. Learning your unique cues and triggers are large steps to being acquainted with yourself. You are no longer running away, but getting comfortable with who you are and how you are.

THE HUNGER SCALE

Let's stop counting what we put into our mouths and tune into our God-given abilities to know when it's time to eat, and when it's time to stop. Bringing balance between neglect and obsession begins with getting into your body and learning what your body requires.

You have built-in hunger and satiety hormones, leptin and ghrelin, and the Holy Spirit to guide you.

The Hunger Scale we will be using is on a 0-5 scale:

0) Empty stomach, feeling hunger pangs, and cues. On the verge of not having self-control. Starving.
1) Ready to eat, hungry, not starving, and able to remain in self-control.
2) Can go another hour or two without eating.
3) Can go another three to four hours without eating.
4) Satisfied. I am comfortable and still have energy.
5) Full. I could have stopped eating 4-5 bites ago and been satisfied.
6) Overfull, lethargic, must unbutton pants or need a nap. I could have stopped eating 10-12 bites ago.

Honoring our hunger and satiety cues is healthy stewardship of our bodies. We don't need to be afraid to eat, nor do we need to be afraid of the inability to stop eating. We will stay between a 1 and 4 on the Hunger Scale, not allowing ourselves to get so hungry we forget to stop eating at satiety. Eating can be an act of worship and an invitation to bring God into all parts of your life. Eating according to the Hunger Scale is about being intentional with your food choices. It can feel uncomfortable at first but will quickly become part of your eating habits.

Get into your body and identify where you are on the Hunger Scale throughout the day.

You are learning lots of new things, so consider using the word "practice" when starting to use the Hunger Scale.

OTHER CONSIDERATIONS

- Eating can be an intentional act of worship.
- Invite the Holy Spirit into your Hunger Scale, food choices, and to the table.
- Eating in the car or standing up can lead to mindless eating.
- Distractions (screens) at the dinner table will prevent you from paying attention to your satiety cues.
- Savor your food and the conversation around the table.
- Certain foods can disrupt your hunger and satiety cues. Pay attention to what brings satiety and what leaves you feeling empty.
- Remember, food is fuel for the body. We are practicing separating using food for emotional needs, and keeping our choices fixed on health.

TIPS

- Dehydration can feel like hunger. Try to drink half your body weight in ounces. (Example: if you are 150 pounds, drink about 75 oz of water).

- Focus on nutrition. Cravings are often a lack of nutrients. Craving chocolate? You might be low in magnesium.

- Skip the sugar. Eating refined sugar skews your hunger and satiety signals and often triggers a binge.

- Balance your plate with protein, a complex carb, and healthy fat to stay satiated.

- Pay attention to portions. Often our eyes are bigger than our stomachs and we initially take more than what is needed to satisfy.

- Have a "crunch at lunch." A great way to beat afternoon snacking and night-time over-eating is adding something crunchy at lunch. Try nuts on your salad, carrots with your sandwich, or celery with your soup.

- Consuming caloric-dense beverages will not help you feel satisfied. Instead choose tea, apple-cider vinegar tonic, lemon water, or naturally flavored seltzers.

- Decrease decision fatigue. Having a meal plan or cycling through 2-5 different options is helpful.

- Food doesn't have to be boring or complicated. Food can be fun, and cooking can be a way to express yourself. Have fun in the kitchen, get your family involved, and try new things!

Please begin to practice and utilize this Hunger Scale throughout your days.

"The righteous has enough to satisfy his appetite…"

Proverbs 13:25

Father, thank You for giving me everything I need for life and godliness and the seal of Your Holy Spirit. You have equipped me to take care of my body, mind, spirit, and emotions. Help me learn these new practices, grant me discernment throughout my day to know what my true hunger is. I won't be able to do this alone, Jesus; I call on your strength and steadfastness to me. Lord, help me tell the difference in my hungers. Please grant me Your full wisdom for my daily choices in taking care of this temple.

2

REMOVE OLD FOUNDATIONS

Investigate Your Ways of Coping and Strengthen
Your Strategy

I LIVED IN AN OLD FARMHOUSE for a few years. It was built in 1890 but had undergone some updating throughout the years. In 1985, the house was raised and a new and larger basement was dug. The foundational walls were strengthened and repaired, along with old footings and pillars. In 2014 when my family moved in, there was nothing for us to do except paint. I didn't have to worry about the walls crumbling, water coming in, mold, or even the spookiness of doing laundry in a 120-year-old basement. The house stood firm, and us within it, because what wasn't strong enough to withstand the elements of life on Earth was replaced. What was not strong enough to keep steady was strengthened and reinforced.

We had to sell our farm a few years later, and when we were in a place to buy another one there was nothing on the market that could compare with the first. None of the basements had been updated; nothing had been reclaimed, restored, or properly maintained so that rot and age didn't take hold. Our sights moved to newer houses with basements still holding strong.

Gaining freedom from emotional eating investigates foundations and asks if they will hold.

We must raise houses (our whole selves), looking underneath to see what may be causing our walls to crack and crumble. We investigate where the wear and tear of our minds have given way for our perceptions to be faulty. We get curious about our coping mechanisms and see if they are healthy and strong enough to hold us up until God calls us home.

It's time to click on the overhead light at the bottom of the stairs and investigate if our thoughts and coping mechanisms will help us withstand what life throws at us. Or if it will crack and crumble, leaving a pile of rubble and a cloud of dust.

We don't do this alone. We go after investigating and repairing with God's help, hand, and strength.

What are your current coping mechanisms? Notice your habits and behaviors of what you run to when under stress.

Have your coping mechanisms led to habits and are now a lifestyle? Do you feel in bondage to them?

Healthy coping strategies will add to your life and health, not subtract.

"For no one can lay a foundation other than the one which is laid, which is Jesus Christ."

1 Corinthians 3:11

"Prepare your work outside and make it ready for yourself in the field, afterwards then build your house." Proverbs 24:27

"By wisdom a house is built, and by understanding it is established; and by knowledge the rooms are filled with all precious and pleasant riches." Proverbs 24:3-4

"The wise woman builds her house, but the foolish plucks it down with her own hands." Proverbs 14:1

LEARN NEW WAYS OF COPING

A Stress Management Plan is Necessary

Webster's Dictionary defines a **coping mechanism** as "any conscious or unconscious adjustment or adaptation that decreases tension and anxiety in a stressful experience or situation."

A **coping strategy** is defined as "an action, a series of actions, or a thought process used in meeting a stressful or unpleasant situation or in modifying one's reaction to a situation. Coping strategies typically involve a conscious and direct approach to problems, in contrast to defense mechanisms."

Emotional eating is a coping mechanism.

We can create a new coping strategy to begin to feel our emotions without being governed or ruled by them. This strategy, or plan, can allow us to live freely in self-control, not using unhealthy mechanisms that lead us to be out of control.

Feeling your emotions and processing them, without eating, is a coping strategy.

The line of whether emotional eating is healthy or not is often determined by the one coping. If it leans into self-harm, self-deprecating and shameful thoughts, it would be an unhealthy coping mechanism.

If emotional eating as a coping mechanism creates a habit, lifestyle, and cycle of bondage, it is unhealthy. If the habit invites disease and destruction to the body, and the rest of one's life, it is unhealthy.

Healthy coping skills are behaviors that we use to make sense of negative experiences productively and positively. They help us manage our emotions related to difficult times to improve emotional health and help us grow as people.

Our middle daughter was born with birth defects resulting in multiple surgeries and a decade of monthly ER visits and ICU stays. I ate my way through five of those ten years, not engaging with the trauma or stress of what was happening to our girl or our family. But it came to a head when I began having panic attacks every time I heard someone cough. I didn't know about trauma, triggers, and coping at the time, and my anxiety stopped going away with food. I had to learn how to cope differently.

Learning healthy coping strategies can take time and often involves trial and error. While looking for what will work, taking a deep breath is a great start.

My healthy coping strategies are:

- Release myself and people from all expectations
- Have quiet/devotional/prayer/processing time each morning
- Give myself space, or taking a time out when emotions/anxiety are high

- Create boundaries for myself around relationships in my life
- Create a weekly food plan and staying with nutrient dense foods
- Make sure I get at least 30 minutes of intentional exercise
- Allow myself to be creative each day (writing, crafting, cooking, etc.)

Planning healthy ways of coping with life is a proactive way of beating emotional eating. Just like having a food plan is important, having a coping plan is essential.

Other ideas for your coping strategy:

- Daily meditation or breath prayer
- Create boundaries for yourself with your time, media, relationships, work/home life, etc.
- Know who to call when you want to isolate or withdraw
- Maintain emotionally supportive relationships
- Ask for help with you need it
- Brain dump your thoughts
- Dance or move your body in a new way
- Have an artistic outlet
- Get in nature, walk, bike, jog, or hike
- Lift weights, take a class at the gym
- Learn a new hobby

Create your strategy or a routine you enjoy.

Create your healthy coping strategy by choosing one thing you will do instead of eat.

Instead of eating emotionally when I feel
_________________ I will _________________.

- Commit to this one strategy, allowing it to become a habit and new way of coping.
- Research other ways of coping and add more items to your coping strategy, implementing them slowly.
- Continue to be proactive and solution-minded, rather than reactive, and see how quickly your stress is lowered and emotions are more easily managed. Having an active coping strategy allows circumstances to remain neutral, and the narrative in your mind to have a way of coping instantly, rather than reaching for one in emotion.

"Do not fear, for I am with you;
Do not be afraid, for I am your God.
I will strengthen you, I will also help you,
I will also uphold you with My righteous
right hand."

Isaiah 41:10

REMOVE OLD THOUGHT PATTERNS

Remove Old Built-Ins and What Does Not Support You

"If you want to change your life, change the way you think." Craig Groeschel

Your thoughts could be the only obstacle between you and your freedom. Thoughts about yourself, your life, your eating habits, and your body could be holding you back. When you have negative emotions or feelings, the first thing you need to do is observe your thoughts. Often, your mind will poke a pain point or trauma, something attached to your emotion, and it will grow. But you can observe your thoughts, rather than become your thoughts.

There are several different thought patterns that emotional eating dips its toe into. Here are two:

Scarcity Mindset: There isn't enough to go around. I'm not enough. It will never be enough. I must hold onto everything because what I have will eventually run out. I must eat all of this now because it won't be available to me later.

Orphan Mindset: I can only rely on myself. People cannot be trusted. Love must be earned. I'm ashamed to ask for help. It's easier to be alone. No one is coming to save me, so

I must save myself. Vulnerability is a sign of weakness.

Both thought patterns are rooted in one thing: fear. Core thoughts that lead to emotional eating can often be reduced to three thought patterns: pride, fear, and shame

There is nothing new under the sun, and as I do more work in this space, I see that the most common denominator to emotional eating is fear. Fear often leads into two directions—pride that says "I can do it on my own, I don't need God or anyone else," and shame that says "Look at what I've done, I'm worthless, helpless, and hopeless."

Both ways of thinking are disempowering, and the opposite of how God wants us to think.

The Bible says God is with us, and our ever-present help. It is written 365 times in the Bible for us not to fear. The Names of God in the Old Testament speak to the characteristics of God as Provider, One Who fights on our behalf, Salvation, Everlasting, Healer, Sanctifier, Peace, Master, Shepherd, and the God of my Righteousness.

How can we begin to work on renewing our minds?

- Write your thoughts or record yourself speaking your stream of consciousness for five minutes.
- Read aloud or listen to the playback.
- Write down all the commands that your thoughts told you about yourself.
- Align them with what the Word says about you, and about God.
- Reject and discard inappropriate and untrue thoughts accordingly.

How to move from scarcity to abundance mindset:

1) Surround yourself with people that add to you and who are "abundance thinkers."
2) Practice gratitude regularly.
3) Look at possibilities rather than mistakes.

How to move from orphaned to Beloved mindset:

1) Get quiet and prayerfully ask the Holy Spirit what ingredients God used, at your creation.
2) Begin reading and speaking out loud the promises of God over your life. You are accepted and not rejected, you are the head and not the tail, etc.
3) Make a list of all the times God has shown up for you in your life, inviting the Holy Spirit to reveal more.

We are not working on fixing the old nature, but coming into our new nature in Christ.

"In reference to your former way of life, you are to rid yourselves of the old self..., and that you are to be renewed in the spirit of your minds, to put on the new self, which in the likeness of God has been created in righteousness and holiness of the truth."

Ephesians 4:22-24

PERFECTIONISM IS FROM THE PIT OF HELL

All-or-nothing thinking likes to classify you and what you do as pass or fail.

When we live with all-or-nothing thoughts, we tend to distort reality, how we interpret events, and how we classify our achievements. All-or-nothing thinking does not allow practice, processes, or errors. It doesn't allow our humanity to be present, like perfectionism. It does not allow you to see growth and will often become a huge boulder in the way of your journey towards food freedom. All-or-nothing thinking is generally bent on the negative and thinks only in absolutes. Rather than thinking in extremes and dwelling on the negative, you can reframe these types of thoughts by choosing to think from a positive perspective. You can choose to see the good, find strength, and understand that setbacks happen, rather than finding faults and giving up entirely.

Let's reframe all-or-nothing thinking with practice and process thoughts.

~

I searched for a while to find a sentence that said this more nicely and still made my point. There wasn't one. Perfectionism is from the pit of hell. I have heard more stories of people being sent into emotional eating or full-blown binges because of one tiny misstep or finding out there was cheese in their "Paleo" soup. Perfectionism is rooted in pride and leads to all-or-nothing thinking and acting.

How many times have you been going along, eating according to plan and one small hiccup sent you into blowing your entire plan for the day, week, month, or year? This may sound extreme, but I have ruined a year's worth of work in weight loss because of one holiday meal. Did I have standards and food rules that were unsustainable? Yes! And holding myself accountable to a standard that was not sustainable kept me in the "on and off the wagon" loop for years. We can jump off the wagon and decide to never climb back on it, but just walk alongside it.

Perfectionism is counterfeit excellence. It reeks of pride, obsession, and bondage. It also smells a lot like fear with the potential of delivering a false identity. What am I if I am not perfect? LOVED. Who am if I am not perfect? HUMAN. To think that you and I will ever be able to reach a standard of perfection is pride and will suck the joy out of living. Perfectionism says, "If it isn't perfect, it isn't good." But God said at our creation that we are "very good." He didn't call us to "be perfect;" God called us to "be fruitful and multiply." We are to be holy as He is Holy, but can only achieve that by faith in Christ.

Thinking you must be perfect is basing your worth on your achievements. This leads to a highly critical inner narrative, with rigid and high expectations of yourself and those around you. This can lead to harmful neglect due to perfectionism's paralyzing nature.

Excellence, on the other hand, is a virtue of goodness. Someone who operates in excellence does their best, expecting nothing more. On some days, my best is much less than someone would expect me to do; on other days it's greater. By removing perfectionism from categorizing yourself and your actions, how does this change your ability to make sustainable choices? Leading life out of a true identity holds space for compassion, kindness, and excellence, not critical standards that lead to more self-harm.

Let's reframe perfectionism, choosing excellence instead.

How often does perfectionism get in the way of you creating new habits in your life?

Write about a time(s) when perfectionism/all-or-nothing thinking were obstacles rather than launching pads for your freedom.

What does perfectionism feel like? What does excellence feel like?

Decide to choose to think and speak in a positive manner about yourself, your life, and those around you.

"Finally, brothers and sisters, whatever is true, whatever is honorable, whatever is right, whatever is pure, whatever is lovely, whatever is commendable, if there is any excellence and if anything, worthy of praise, think about these things. As for the things you have learned and received and heard and seen in me, practice these things, and the God of peace will be with you."

Philippians 4:8-9

COUNTERFEIT FREEDOM

Freedom Gained Your Own Way May Not Be True Freedom

A person who is trained to identify a counterfeit bill does not study counterfeit bills. The person studies a real bill to the point of knowing it so thoroughly that he or she can spot even the best counterfeit.

The weight and thickness of the paper.

The ink pigments, colors, and even color-shifting ink.

Watermarks, security threads, microprinting, serial numbering.

And so much more.

The investigator's doubt and lack of faith in the counterfeit can only be as strong as their attention to the details of the truth. We are to do the same with the Word of God, to not be caught off guard or entangled by distractions from the enemy. Anything the enemy offers us is a counterfeit. Anything the world offers us with the belief that we can have freedom in life independent from God is counterfeit.

We have believed that following a diet perfectly or getting to a certain weight will save us somehow. But after we take the bait, thinking it is the way out, we find ourselves in more entrapment looking for another way out.

Have you thought: "This will be the diet to fix me. This will be the way out of my overweight body, and I will be able to follow and keep it off for life. I will start tomorrow and make perfect choices from here on out, so I'm going to eat all this stuff now. This food will make me feel better. This diet will fix all my issues."

What are some counterfeits you have bought into? What lies have you believed about yourself, your body, and weight loss?

What rules have you picked up and believed are necessary for weight loss?

Why are they counterfeit?

Counterfeit freedom is anything you do or believe to be "the way" that is independent of God. Maybe this whole time you have been working on dieting, losing weight, overcoming emotional eating, and have done it separately or independently from God. Have you believed that it's up to you to get it right?

What if this is a new place in your life where God wants to show Himself faithful to you, and mighty to what you battle?

You don't have to do this alone and you get to pull on heavenly power to take down what may be a giant of emotional eating. If overcoming eating is a heavy weight you are carrying, decide to drop it and roll it over to the Lord.

I am so grateful that I was not able to get free on my own. I would have dipped into pride that would not be pleasing to the Lord. But He has been so gracious to me, in teaching me, that it is "not by power, nor by might, but by the Spirit of God." (Zechariah 4:6).

- What are you currently doing on your own, with your eating patterns or ways of getting free from food?
- What rules, habits, and mindsets have been built around food that is independent of God?
- What is the Holy Spirit asking you to believe about God and how He wants to take you into freedom?
- What counterfeit freedom are you letting go of today, because it is independent of doing this God's way?

"No temptation has overtaken you except something common to mankind, and God is faithful, so He will not allow you to be tempted beyond what you are able, but with the temptation will provide the way of escape also, so that you will be able to endure it."

1 Corinthians 10:13

3

REFRAME YOUR WHY

Your Reason for Freedom is About More Than You Think

IN ATTEMPTING TO LOSE THE WEIGHT I gained during emotional/binge eating, I signed up for every diet program known to man. Each program started the same way: identify your "why" for losing weight. Determining "my why" felt like an after-thought and my answer was always "I'm overweight and I don't want to be." But just as dieting does not help emotional eating, wanting to lose weight never helped me lose it. Perhaps because I tend to go deeper into everything, shallow "whys" only offered shallow change. We must get to the root of why we are doing what we are doing, or our hearts simply won't be in it.

I hope by now you understand this book is not about a diet program or written for weight loss. We must heal our emotional eating before attempting to lose weight, or the cycle will continue. There are hundreds of different ways you can lose weight, but only one way to gain victory over emotional eating: heal.

Remove weight loss from your Why.

When we reframe something in our mind, we are choosing to see it a different way. I want you to understand so badly that you are more than your body and more than your eating habits. I want you to understand that what you eat and how much you weigh have nothing to do with your value or worth. They are simply measurements of a thing that is under the pull of gravity. People might value what we look like, but God has already called us His Image-Bearers. He values who we are, not what we do or how we look.

> *"...For God does not see as man*
> *sees, since man looks at the*
> *outward appearance, but the Lord*
> *looks at the heart."*
>
> *1 Samuel 16:7*

My goal in *Food Freedom* is for you to understand your value and worth, in Christ, thereby giving you the tenacity to stop using food as a coping tool forever. You have a purpose for being here, a calling to walk in, and advancing the Kingdom of God is part of it. The enemy would like nothing more than for you to not realize who you are, and get you to believe that your struggle with food is an obstacle to your purpose and calling.

Do you have thoughts like:

"How could I ever start a ministry when I can't control myself at the dessert table?"

"How can I lay hands on the sick when I have no control over the simplest thing—eating?"

"I will write that book, get that degree, start that ministry, become a missionary, etc. when I lose the weight."

How sly the enemy is to use something God gave us—food—to contort our relationship with God, and become a barrier to advancing His Kingdom.

Food has been used:

- against us
- to control us
- to berate us
- to keep us in bondage to it
- to keep us held back from moving God's Kingdom forward

When I realized this, I got angry.

Not only was my struggle with eating a cover-up to my pain, it was used against me in full deception. My "why" quickly changed from weight loss to shoving my victory over food in the face of the enemy.

"As for you, you meant evil against me, but God meant it for good to bring about this present result, to keep many people alive."

Genesis 50:20

When this revelation came to me in 2018, I was determined to never let food, or my body, define me again—those false identities are dead and buried in the grave. Emotional eating robs us. It robs us of inviting the presence of God into our pain. It creates a chasm between what we feel and what we value.

Looking back on 36 years of emotional eating, not only was my health stolen, but so were years of peace, joy, fulfillment, and some relationships. I couldn't see beyond the binge or defeat each time I gave in. Emotional eating can snuff out the seeds of faith that have been planted within you.

- What has emotional eating stolen from you?
- What do you want to declare today that is dead in the grave, and no longer has power over you or your food choices?
- What has God already spoken to you about your healing and freedom from food?
- In your food choices, what is God asking you to surrender to Him?

"The thief comes only to kill, steal and destroy, but I have come [Jesus said] to give you life, and life abundant."

John 10:10

"Therefore, if anyone is in Christ, this person is a new creation; the old things passed away; behold, new things have come."

2 Corinthians 5:17

CULTIVATE YOUR WHY

Determine Your Values, Not Just Your Vision

Shallow "whys" will get us nowhere except shallow and short-lived change. To root down and cultivate your Why, you must determine your values. Our self-sabotage and self-harm keep us locked down in a spiral after we overeat because we went against a value. I value personal freedom, health, honesty, hope, ability, work ethic, and creativity; in my patterns of emotional eating, most of my values were compromised. This is why I felt shame, and the enemy made my failure a party. Compromising our values fragments parts of our character. We can feel that we've lost a part of ourselves, and we may never get it back, the further down the hole of addiction or bondage we go.

A lot of our frustration with ourselves could be because we are not living as who we truly are.

By putting our values back in sight, realigning with them, and creating an action plan according to them, we can root down change and cultivate the life we want to live.

A value is a set of beliefs, priorities, or views that we find most important in our lives. Values affect the way we act and make decisions. Determining our values will bring things into focus and make our reasons clearer.

To find your values, here are some questions to help you reflect and identify them:

- What time in your life have you been happiest?
- When have you felt most fulfilled or proud?
- What time in your life have you struggled with the most?
- Who do you admire most?
- What is on your bucket list?
- What do you hope other people describe you as when you're not around?
- What habits do you want to build?
- Do you have an inherited value, something passed down in your family?
- What scriptures do you value that can help you unlock one of yours?
- What attributes of God do you value?

Find themes or connections that help determine your values.

Write your values, and to further support them, write why they are your values. (You can do a series of 5-7 whys to find the root of why these are your values.)

"He has told you, mortal one,
what is good;
And what does the LORD
require of you
But to do justice, to love
kindness,
And to walk humbly with your
God?"

Micah 6:8

REBUILD YOUR WHY

Write the Vision for Your Victory Based on Values

Scripture tells us we are co-heirs and co-creators with Christ. And since "God so loved the world that He gave His One and Only Son," (John 3:16), we understand that relationship is a value of God. I believe God wants to show us so much more of Who He is and His Kingdom, that His Holy Spirit waits patiently, yet zealously, for us to understand.

There is a last day in your lifetime when you will stop emotionally eating. It could be today, next month, a year from now, or the day you go home to Jesus. Whenever that last day is, even as you read this, you are already free. Galatians 5:1 states, "it is for freedom that Christ has set us free, therefore do not submit again to the yoke of slavery." God already sees you free because Jesus has set you free. You are just fleshing this freedom out in your mortal body through thoughts and actions.

God is future-focused, and His mercies are new each morning (Lamentations 3:22).

Since your Why is no longer attached to weight loss, and is now attached to your values, let's begin to recognize and create the vision for your life.

In the last chapter, one of the questions you were to answer was "what ingredients did God put into you, at your creation?" Please pull out your answers and combine them with your values.

- Take a deep breath, close your eyes, and prayerfully ask the Holy Spirit to show you why your victory over food is necessary for the Kingdom of God.
- Go on a journey, record what you see, what you hear, and what God shows you. If you want to talk through it, rather than write, record the audio of what you are shown.

Because your life is not your own and is so much bigger than you, dreaming and vision-casting with God is monumental.

- What are you supposed to do on this earth?
- Who are the people you have you been called to?
- How does God want you to walk out this life?
- How do your ingredients and values play into your calling?
- Why does the enemy use food to attempt to steal your life away?
- Why is it so important for you to steward the temple of the Holy Spirit well?

*"I will stand at my guard post
And station myself on the
watchtower;
And I will keep watch to see what
He will say to me,
And how I may reply when I am
reprimanded.
Then the LORD answered me and
said,
"Write down the vision
And inscribe it clearly on tablets,
So that one who reads it may run.
For the vision is yet for the
appointed time;
It hurries toward the goal and it
will not fail.
Though it delays, wait for it;
For it will certainly come, it will not
delay long."*

Habakkuk 2:1-4

God also values obedience. The Old Testament is full of sacrifices made on behalf of people who were disobedient to the Law of God—Enter Jesus, the perfect and final sacrifice.

"Does the LORD have as much delight in
burnt offerings and sacrifices
As in obeying the voice of the LORD?
Behold, to obey is better than a sacrifice,
And to pay attention is better than the
fat of rams."

1 Samuel 15:22

Not only did Christ live a sacrificial life to His death, He did so in heart of obedience because of His love for the Father. The Hebrew word "šāma" is used in this scripture for "obey" or "obeying." It means to listen, understand, declare, discern, obey, and witness. It is the same word used when Adam and Eve were walking in the garden and heard the voice of the Lord. It is the same word used when God spoke to Abraham, to the people of Israel, and all throughout the Old Testament.

In the New Testament we learn through the example of Jesus, believers *are called to a life of obedience*, which can also translate to

- Trust
- Hear and Act
- Submit and Surrender

Jesus calls us to obey out of our love for Him.

"If you love Me, you will keep My commandments."

John 14:15

Obedience is an act of worship.

"Therefore, I urge you, brothers and sisters, by the mercies of God, to present your bodies as a living and holy sacrifice, acceptable to God, which is your spiritual service of worship."

Romans 12:1

Most of moving from defeat to victory, in food freedom, is being aware of what/who you are being obedient to. We can be obedient to things that are not for our good or become obedient to the higher calling that God has on our lives.

After the Holy Spirit and I went on the value and vision journey that you just did, I was stumped. What I saw was a glimpse of a life that I was not living at the time, nor could I achieve on my own. No manipulation or creation of mine would get me to where I am to be. Only by closely following the voice of God, and being obedient to Him, would I ever be able to fulfill the plan He has for my life.

Victory in food freedom is attained the same way; it is year by year, month by month, day by day, choice by choice. It does not happen overnight, but after faithfully walking in obedience to the voice of God, you will find yourself there one day.

What is holding you back from obeying your own values?

Have you been living in sacrifice rather than obedience?

Is there a part of you that is rebellious and does not want to obey what the Lord is speaking to you about your eating habits? Why?

Name one thing and put into practice your act of obedience to the Lord.

> *"Whenever God's will is in the ascendant, all compulsion is gone. When we choose deliberately to obey Him, then He will tax the remotest star and the last grain of sand to assist us with all His almighty power." -Oswald Chambers*

REBUILD WALLS OF STEWARDSHIP AND SURRENDER

Being temples of the Holy Spirit and coming into fully trusting the Lord, we get to steward our bodies in health, then surrender them back to the Lord.

Stewardship is taking on the responsibility of what God has given us. We steward our time, our finances, our relationships. We steward and train up our children. We steward businesses and the people who work for us. Stewardship is hard and can be done in ungodly or godly ways. Since we house the Holy Spirit, we are to take responsibility for where He dwells and abides.

Stewarding begs for us to look at our lives as God-focused and future-thinking.

Stewardship:

- Is not driven by impulse or feelings
- Rises above emotions
- Comes to a higher standard of thinking, living, and acting
- Makes choices according to values, not worldly standards
- Is a well-balanced mindset that leads to total wellness

Stewardship is taking responsibility for our relationship with God, putting our emotions in a place where they are honored but are not governing us. It also dissolves thoughts that do not line up with what God says. In food freedom, stewardship is choosing health over comfort, which leads to greater self-control. You are the temple of the Holy Spirit. Being that God's Spirit lives inside of you, you can ask Him how to best take care of His house, and He will answer.

Emotional hunger only thinks about right now, while stewardship looks at the whole picture.

Emotional hunger says, "I need comfort right now! Therefore, I will eat!"

Stewardship says, "God is the only source of true comfort. Therefore, I will pray for His comfort."

God does not call us to run to anything other than Him, our refuge. He does not tell us to escape, hide, and numb our feelings. He calls us to Himself, calling us higher to do things His way. It is often a calling of exercising our faith amidst the chaos, confusion, and circumstances that surround us. His grace allows us to stand with His strength.

Surrender is not one of the most appealing ideas in the 21ˢᵗ century, let alone submission or yielding.

When God places His finger on something in our lives, good or bad, that He wants us to give up or surrender over to Him, it is for our good and His glory. Often, what He asks us to surrender is something that is killing us or keeping us from His best.

Sometimes the conviction comes like a thunderbolt down from heaven that we are thinking, doing, or using something that could harm us. The Holy Spirit reveals it to us, and with God's strength, we can drop it. We can see what wasn't good for us, and with quick obedience turn it over.

Other times, the Holy Spirit will woo us to surrender something over to the Lord, and we wrestle. We cannot see all the good things that are on the other side of surrender. But as the Lord has already shown you what He has in store for your life, you can surrender in gratitude and excitement.

- Has God been asking you, or wooing you, to take a break from something?
- What in your life is the Holy Spirit asking you to surrender?
- What ideas, thoughts, old agreements, or false identities is God asking you to surrender to Him?
- Why is God putting His finger on these things?
- What is God asking you to pick up in stewardship of your body and emotions?

*"The one who is faithful in a very
little thing is also faithful in much."*

Luke 16:10

REMOVE HEAVY YOKES

It is recorded in Matthew 11:28-30 that Jesus said "Come to Me, all who are weary and burdened, and I will give you rest. Take My yoke upon you and learn from Me, for I am gentle and humble in heart, and *you will find rest for your souls.* For My yoke is comfortable, and My burden is light."

The heaviness of carrying whatever you have been carrying must be taxing and weighing on you. I didn't know how heavy my burdens and yokes were until I wasn't carrying them anymore.

Jesus doesn't see us carrying these yokes of bondage and shoo us away. He doesn't say "clean yourself up first, then I will deal with you." No, Jesus says "come to Me, all of you who are weary and burdened, and I will give you rest."

Are you looking for rest from carrying these habits and feelings of defeat? You can drop them at the feet of Jesus. For us to take on the light and easy yoke of Christ, we must first remove the yokes that are heavy and burdensome. We must remove the yokes of slavery to food or comfort. We must dethrone our ways of doing things, and our ways of "handling it."

We must uproot what means to take us down and out in life, and take up the yoke of Christ that helps us walk in freedom. Throughout your life, pay attention if heaviness is trying to come upon you, and ask the Holy Spirit to identify what it is. When we take off yokes that we are not to carry, sometimes our mind thinks they are our "job." But as Jesus has said, our job is to come and lay them down, and only carry what He tells us to carry.

- What heavy emotions is the Lord asking you to give to Him today?
- What yokes and ways of doing things are you ready to lay down today?
- What has diet culture taught you about taking care of your body that is too heavy to bear?
- How is the Holy Spirit inviting you into rest with your food freedom?

"Are you weary, carrying a heavy burden? Come to me. I will refresh your life, for I am your oasis. Simply join your life with mine. Learn my ways and you'll discover that I'm gentle, humble, easy to please. You will find refreshment and rest in me. For all that I require of you will be pleasant and easy to bear."
Matthew 11:28-30 TPT

"Are you tired? Worn out? Burned out on religion? Come to me. Get away with me and you'll recover your life. I'll show you how to take a real rest. Walk with me and work with me—watch how I do it. Learn the unforced rhythms of grace. I won't lay anything heavy or ill-fitting on you. Keep company with me and you'll learn to live freely and lightly." Matthew 11:28-30 MSG

VISUALIZE YOUR FOOD FREEDOM

Imagine yourself fully walking in food freedom and record how your life has changed:

- What does it feel like to live in self-control, and not afraid of losing control with food?
- How do you live in your body differently now that you are free?
- How are your finances?
- How has your relationship with God changed?
- How have other relationships in your life changed?
- Describe your new normal.
- What does freedom eating look like?
- What are your habits?

- How do you act around holidays, birthdays, celebrations, and stressful situations?
- Fully visualize your life in food freedom, 6 months, 12 months, and 5 years from now.

What emotions do you feel when you see yourself living fully free from food? Record 3-5 emotions that you will feel when you are walking fully in victory.

FACE YOUR WHY NOT

You have visualized what your life will look like walking in full freedom. You have seen the big plans God has for your life, your purpose, and calling. You have witnessed yourself living fully free from food.

And now we need to flip the tables.

Visualize what your life looks like remaining in bondage and still living in emotional eating. Imagine yourself and your life remaining bound, chained, and not free.

- What does it feel like and look like to be in your body?
- What does it feel like to not have self-control, still afraid of food?
- What does your body look like? How does your body feel, still recovering from binging or emotional eating?
- How are your finances?
- How is your relationship with God changed?
- How have other relationships changed in your life?
- Describe your daily life. What are you eating? What are your habits? How do you act around holidays, birthdays, celebrations, and stressful situations?

Fully visualize your life still in bondage and not free from food, 6 months, 12 months, and 5 years from now.

What are the 3-5 emotions that you feel while visualizing your life still in defeat and not walking in victory?

CREATE YOUR FOOD FREEDOM WHY

After doing the heavy work of visualizing your life free and not free from food, we get to create your foundational statement for doing this work.

I imagine emotions emerged while you did these exercises, and you felt a string of different senses.

Did your freedom feel like some of the fruits of the Spirit?

Love? Joy? Peace? Patience? Kindness? Gentleness? Goodness? Self-control?

When you flipped the tables, what was waiting?

Fear? Frustration? Hopelessness? Helplessness? More Defeat?

Knowing and remaining true to your values can help you move the needle towards your food freedom. They remind you, and tell the world, who you are, what you will and will not stand for. They are a standard that you have placed upon yourself. Often when you don't feel you are living in agreement with your values, you feel that you have let yourself down or are not living to your full potential.

Create your *Food Freedom* Why statement from answering these questions:

- Why do you want to get and stay free?
- Why are your values more important than just losing weight or being at a certain size?
- What are the bigger picture and bigger reasons for you getting free from food and emotional eating?
- What is at stake if you do not put in the work to fully step into your God-given freedom?
- How does your food freedom impact those around you?

Put it all together in paragraph form. Your *Food Freedom* Why is an essential part of creating your lasting freedom plan and moving into all that God has for you in life.

> *"Now the Lord is the Spirit, and where the Spirit of the Lord is, there is freedom." 2 Corinthians 3:17*

> *"For those who are according to the flesh set their minds on the things of the flesh, but those who are according to the Spirit, the things of the Spirit."*

> *Romans 8:5*

4

RECOGNIZE PATTERNS

Come Out of Autopilot and Come into Awareness

EMOTIONAL EATING OFTEN COMES from a place of autopilot. Since we have learned this way of coping, the brain will tap into what it's always done when an emotion arises—because that is what it has always done. In this chapter you will learn how to recognize a few things:

- Patterns of emotions and your way of coping
- Patterns of eating that you may be aware of, but are unaware of why you participate in them
- The Holy Spirit speaking to you throughout your day and in your choices

Before we begin, I want to make one thing clear: nowhere during your healing journey are you allowed to judge yourself. We will look at your emotions and patterns objectively, but not judge them, or yourself. We are all starting today and acknowledging that God longs to meet you right where you are. In your life, you are meant for freedom, health, and wholeness, and this is just the heavy lifting we must do to get you there.

God's plan and purpose will always be to draw you to Himself in intimacy and He just may use your eating to do so. You don't get to decide if you are good or bad, because it's already been decided and spoken into fruition at your creation: you are VERY GOOD.

First, define what a binge or emotional eating episode is to you.

Clinically, a binge is defined as consuming more than 1500 calories above your total daily need. A binge to me, or an emotional eating episode, would be anything I eat when I am using food for emotional reasons: to numb, escape, not feel, run, or fall into self-pity with the mindset of "I may as well eat." I used to often do it in boredom, fear, or just habit. A binge or emotional eating can be described as eating when not hungry because emotional hunger and physical hunger are separate.

What does binge/emotional eating look like for you? What are the patterns of emotional eating that you participate in?

Since awareness is the first step to change, it is helpful to describe your pattern as detailed as you can.

- What do you do?
- Why do you do it?
- When do you do it?
- What is the pattern while you are emotionally eating?
- What is the trigger?
- Do you have an emotional trigger and a food-related trigger?
- What are the emotions you feel before you head into a binge/episode? What do they have in common?
- What foods trigger you to binge? List the feelings that they produce in you.
- What other things do you notice about your emotional eating pattern?

"For in him we live and move and have our being. As some of your own poets have said, 'We are his offspring.'"

Acts 17:28

INSERTING YOURSELF BETWEEN STIMULUS AND RESPONSE

Come Out of Reacting and Into Responding

Emotional eating is the physical form of emotional stuffing, so we must begin to feel our feelings to stop stuffing. To do this, we learn how to insert ourselves between our circumstances and our responses to those circumstances.

> *"Between stimulus and response there is a space. In that space is our power to choose our response. In our response lies our growth and our freedom."*
>
> *Viktor Frankl*

We all have circumstances (stimulus) surrounding us. These circumstances are neutral. They have no voice or memory, they simply are. A truly neutral circumstance can be proven in a court of law with multiple witnesses.

For example:

Circumstance/Stimulus: My daughter asked for a store-bought birthday cake, rather than homemade.

Anyone around us during this conversation could tell you this exact circumstance because this is what she said; it is a fact.

My response to her statement is where I get to decide how to react. I could react and allow my thoughts to fly one hundred miles per hour, hitting pain point after pain point in my brain:

"She doesn't want a homemade cake because I'm a terrible baker."

"She asked for store-bought because I can't decorate like a professional and it's embarrassing."

"She's afraid I will screw up her cake and therefore mess up her entire party. I can't do anything right."

And on and on.

I could choose to lean into an interpretation that is hurtful for me to think and feel, or I could remain neutral in my response. My daughter was not trying to hurt me at all, but I could be hurt by my interpretation of what she said.

Instead, I remain neutral and ask, "Would you like chocolate or vanilla, and which store would you like it from?"

This is where we get to choose our response and where our freedom lives, remaining neutral in our response. There is no emotion in neutrality. I don't allow my thoughts to go flying, I don't assume or get myself worked up. I can learn to remain neutral emotionally by focusing on the circumstance and reality at hand, and my response to it. I can either make it really big in my mind and heart or keep it neutral.

Take a breath, get into your body, and create a space between the circumstance and your reaction, so that you can respond with wisdom and remain neutral. You will find certain circumstances may hit pain points or trigger your emotions, but look at the facts of the situation, and choose your response accordingly. This takes time and practice. You can also work on your body language and tone of voice while you practice your response.

By the way, I talked with my daughter about the store-bought cake. She didn't want me to stress about making one.

~

It's good to remain as neutral as possible, not like a wall of stone, but non-reactionary. Since we always have a narrative playing in our minds, we can control the emotional charge by sticking to the circumstances and the facts. This is a way to create a mental and emotional boundary for yourself, choosing your interpretation.

It is often what we think and how we internalize the thought that hurts us. We often get hurt by people because we misinterpret their words or actions and react out of our pain. We then turn towards more self-harm— emotional eating. Take the time to think better. When we recognize patterns of ourselves getting "worked up" over something neutral, this can help us come down quicker.

A few healthy response tips:

- Step out of the room/situation to collect your thoughts and come out of your feelings.
- Put the phone down after receiving a hurtful text and come out of your feelings before responding.
- Acknowledge your feelings before going into a stressful situation and create a plan to decompress later.

- Create mental/emotional boundaries by not allowing things/people to upset you (i.e. "my emotions are mine and are not governed by my circumstances or someone else's feelings. I can remain stable, unwavering and stand unaffected by my circumstance.")

At the end of the day, you are not responsible for the circumstances around you; you are responsible for your response to them. I have often walked into triggering and volatile situations and needed to decompress and debrief for a few days after. It would make the circumstance worse if I added emotional eating to it.

Allow yourself the time to respond well and neutrally.

Prayerfully create healthy boundaries for yourself to not take on someone else's emotions (I call this Holy Spirt Teflon).

Recognize patterns/people that add or subtract to your life and create appropriate boundaries.

Create a plan for how you will respond in high-stress situations and put it into practice.

Allow yourself to feel when you are in a safe space and talk things out with a trusted friend/counselor.

Do not allow someone/something outside of yourself to cause you to self-harm.

"Finally, brothers and sisters, whatever is true, whatever is honorable, whatever is right, whatever is pure, whatever is lovely, whatever is commendable, if there is any excellence and if anything, worthy of praise, think about these things. As for the things you have learned and received and heard and seen in me, practice these things, and the God of peace will be with you."

Philippians 4:8-9

EMOTIONAL EATING AT ITS CORE

Identify Your Core Fear and Remove the Enemy's Easy Button

At the base of all sin or taking things into our own hands are three common themes: pride, shame, and fear.

Pride says we don't need God; we think we are higher than God.

Shame says there is something wrong with us at our core. We are not enough, and we are already handcuffed and condemned.

Fear comes in many forms. At the base of most fears, being alone is the most common: fear of rejection, abandonment, failure, success, etc.

These three are Satan's playground. Since he cannot create, but only imitate God, the devil twists and contorts our reasons to make them feel right and okay to us, all the while keeping us from God's best. When our reasons are contorted, our identity comes under fire and our intimacy with God is at stake.

Finding out your core fear can give you a superpower. When I found mine, fear of abandonment, I leveled up towards my food freedom.

The enemy knew that pushing my "abandonment button" was all he had to do to send me flying to the pantry. I can imagine, as in *The Screwtape Letters*, the enemy plotting for my demise. "Just get her to believe that people are mad at her. Get her to think that her husband is cheating or going to leave her. Get her to believe that her kids will die or grow up and leave her. Get her to believe that God has left her because she has screwed up so many times. Get her to believe that she is alone, and no one is coming to help her."

One poke, one triggering thought, was all the enemy needed to take me down.

It was the same trigger as when I was a kid. "No one is coming, and I am alone."

I noticed my patterns of eating when my husband left on a work trip, when I was in conflict with a friend or family member, or when I felt overwhelmed.

Once we notice a pattern and find our core fear, we can investigate further and have a leg up on the enemy and our autopilot. The deeper you can go with answering the questions, the more awareness and freedom you will achieve.

Knowing what you do and why you do it is a superpower that not many people can tap into or wield.

Invite the Holy Spirit into questioning your habits and patterns. Ask God for wisdom; He will surely provide.

"My child, if you will receive
my words
And treasure my
commandments within you,
Make your ear attentive to
wisdom;
Incline your heart to
understanding.
For if you cry out for insight,
And raise your voice for
understanding;
If you seek her as silver
And search for her as for
hidden treasures;
Then you will understand the
fear of the Lord,
And discover the knowledge of
God."

Proverbs 2:1-5

AWARENESS OF CONSEQUENCES

Recognize How Binge or Emotional Eating Affects You Wholly

Since emotional eating is a "right now," once we become aware of the pattern it is easier to identify when we are heading into another cycle. By turning off autopilot in our decisions with food, we can live one or two steps ahead of our choices. How do we turn off our autopilot? We must become aware of our thoughts and understand our thoughts are not 100% truth. They are just thoughts. The enemy likes to twist our thoughts by feeding us half-truths or full-on lies. By creating a thought pattern of "I have no power over food," and by living out this thought by our actions, affirming a belief, a bondage is created.

Bondage wants you to believe that it is the only choice you have. It wants you to believe that you have no choice in what you do, except to continue to choose "it." Our auto-pilot responses to the circumstances of life can cause triggers that create a circumstance for us to exercise our God-given free will. This exercising or practice is based on coming out of that autopilot, or limbic system, and stepping into consciousness. We can make choices for our lives in a peaceful, responsive way, instead of reacting in haste. Freedom lays out many choices for you, like an unhurried buffet.

"My son, pay attention to my wisdom,
Incline your ear to my understanding,
So that you may maintain discretion
And your lips may comply with
knowledge.
For the lips of an adulteress drip honey,
And her speech is smoother than oil;
But in the end she is bitter as wormwood,
Sharp as a two-edged sword.
Her feet go down to death,
Her steps take hold of Sheol.
She does not ponder the path of life;
Her ways are unstable, she does not
know it."

Proverbs are full of contrasting choices between wisdom and foolishness. We are taught that we must look closely at what is being offered to us, because foolishness often mirrors, but mocks, wisdom. Proverbs 5 explains that to gain wisdom, we must turn our focus and listen for understanding. That's a big difference from just hearing. We must focus and pay attention to gain and maintain maturity. We do this so that what we say and do are in accordance with what we know: wisdom is knowledge applied. The adulteress or the thing that will take mislead us sounds sweet and feels easy, but in the end is just bitterness. We will be hurt by following its bait.

The Holy Spirit guided me to sit and look closer at a few lines from this scripture.

"Her feet go down to death." Her feet are the base of her choice. We must look at where our choices are rooted. We must see what is beyond the immediate need, because every choice we make will plant or water a seed.

"Her steps take hold of Sheol." We can become aware of the consequences of our choices if they are heaven or hell-bound. We must ask ourselves, "Where will this choice take me; where will I be headed?"

"She does not ponder the path of life; her ways are unstable; she does not know it." The path of the one that is not a forward thinker, or someone who looks at the repercussions of their choices beforehand, is unstable and only living moment to moment, going nowhere.

We must investigate where our choices are rooted to see the outcome before it happens. If they are rooted in fear, pride, or shame we know they are hell-bound. When we live on autopilot, we aren't thinking "Where is this headed?" We are only thinking of quelling the immediate need of our uncomfortable emotions at the time.

How many times, after a binge or an emotional eating episode, have you asked yourself "Why did I do that?" or "How could I have blown it that bad?"

You lost control, you were only thinking and feeling in the moment, not thinking about how you would feel afterward. Part of awareness is having the forethought to ask, "Where will this take me?" And that's how we can turn our past "failures" into lessons so that we will know better for next time.

After a binge—an hour, or the next day—I would feel terrible emotionally, mentally, physically, and spiritually.

Emotionally, I was tanked and I felt worse than I did before I started overeating. Not only was the anxiety or feeling still there, it was amplified by shame and frustration. Fear was also magnified because I was searching for a way to "fix" what I had done to my body.

Mentally, I was foggy because the food I ate brought brain fog. I was unable to make good decisions for the rest of the day and into the next day. I had no self-confidence that I would be able to make it through the day without again.

Physically, I was bloated, lethargic, my joints hurt, and old injuries were more prominent. My digestion was always messed up and often took 2-4 days to get back to normal patterns. I usually put on 6-10 pounds of weight, 1-3 of those pounds being actual fat, the rest being inflammation and water.

Spiritually, I felt distant from God, often ashamed of what I had done because I knew better. I had blown a perfectly good opportunity for me to rest and rely on God. Instead I chose to numb out and seek a counterfeit comfort.

A momentary feeling, that could have lasted 5 minutes if I dealt with it appropriately, resulted in three to four days' worth of consequences.

Not the mention the neural pathways in my brain to binge were reinforced, rather than the new pathways I was working to create.

The voice of the one tempting me away was sweet and smooth. "There, there, dear. This will make you feel better." But choosing that way only led to a personal hell.

Let's look at the true nature and outcome of your emotional eating pattern, but remember these are just behaviors and are not attached to who you are.

Take a deep breath, close your eyes. Go back to your last binge, or a time when emotional eating was taking place. Invite the Holy Spirit to show you:

- How did it start? What was the trigger?
- What was the thought pattern, or what were you feeling?
- Name all the things you ate, and if you can, write down your thoughts as you ate.
- What were you numbing or running from?
- When it was over, what did you feel emotionally?
- When it was over, what were you thinking about?
- Did you feel closer or more distant from God?
- How did it feel in your body? How did your stomach feel? How did it feel to breathe?
- The day after, how did you feel emotionally, mentally, spiritually, and physically?

Be as detailed as you can in your description and allow truth in love to move in and through you.

- How has your perspective about this pattern changed?
- Is part of your frustration due to not living according to your personal values?
- Read Psalm 139.

"God is spirit, and his worshipers must worship in the Spirit and in truth."

John 4:24

"Then you will know the truth, and the truth will set you free."

John 8:32

"Now the Lord is the Spirit, and where the Spirit of the Lord is, there is freedom."

2 Corinthians 3:17

Lord, You see me and You know me even more intimately than I know myself. You know my thoughts before I think them, and my words before I speak them. You know my coming in and my going out. You know why I do the things that I do, and You do not shame me for them, but call me higher. Holy Spirit, lead me into all truth, for it is Jesus and Jesus alone that can satisfy.

AWARENESS OF ABIDING WISDOM WITHIN YOU

Find God in your Choices and Lean on His Strength

You don't have to do this on your own.

You don't have to figure out how to get free, especially once you realize that you already are free in Christ.

The Holy Spirit is Helper and Comforter, so let's invite Him into those places where we need help and comfort the most.

When I started inviting God into my food choices, I was afraid it would be salads for days and shame when I didn't choose to listen to Him first, but that was not my experience.

Inviting God into your meals, food plan, and into your feelings brings us to a place of intimacy that we have been longing for. He is an ever-present help, and His wisdom will point us directly to what our bodies and souls need. And really, God is fun.

As we come out of years of body obsession, diet-cycling, and fear-based eating patterns, rest and peace are waiting for us.

For years, I was on a low-calorie diet, restricting carbohydrates down to a bare minimum and physically running myself ragged. When I was asked, "Are you free and are you being kind to yourself?" my answer was a resounding "NO!" I started to investigate where my habits and patterns had gone from one ditch of neglect into the other ditch of obsession. Being neither free nor kind to myself, I had to allow the Holy Spirit to advise me because I knew the world would not help. The Holy Spirit led me toward disciplined freedom. My boundaries did not become looser but turned to glorify God.

I asked, "Lord what should I have for breakfast?" and He answered me.

I asked, "Lord what should I have for lunch?" and He answered me.

I asked, "Lord what should I have for dinner?" and He answered me in a way I didn't expect: "Add a potato."

The body calls for certain nutrients, vitamins, and minerals that we get from food. If the body is calling for protein and we feed it carbs, the body will still call (or send a craving) for protein. On a smaller level, if the body is running low on magnesium and it hormonally sends a craving to our brain, if we are not "listening" or "in-tune" we may feed it what it is not calling for; and the cycle of craving starts again. God made our bodies magnificent and wonderful.

Your body is designed to work for you—it is your job to listen to it.

We were also designed to listen to the Holy Spirit and allow Him to guide our choices.

In my healing journey, I have been led in disciplined freedom. This looks like eating in a way that fuels my activity and nourishes my body, not invoking inflammation or other health issues. Once or twice per week, I have dessert and I enjoy it fully.

If you were around to hear my kids talk about my eating habits, you would hear, "Mom only eats healthy. Mom doesn't eat sugar. Mom always gets a salad instead of pizza." But that's only half of the picture. My kids didn't see me in the pantry or the times that I was face deep in their boxes of cereal and lunchbox potato chips because I couldn't resist anymore. I did more damage living in restriction than I would have done living in balance.

In my "why," I state that "I want to be a normal eater."

Normal to me is:

- Able to say "no" without regret or restriction
- Not in an emotional relationship with food
- Being a person that viewed food rightly; a neutral thing that couldn't ever love me back.
- Able to create a food plan that reflected healthy living, but also balance.

I was led on many occasions to say "yes" to eating things that my discipline would have otherwise said "no." I began to say "yes" to eating one or two cookies that my ten-year-old daughter made, without fear that I would lose control. And they were the best cookies I ever had.

I was led to make and enjoy Sunday desserts, like my once-famous Peach Plus Pie. Other times, I was led to pass on the birthday cake that didn't belong to someone I deeply loved, and to forgo the dessert table at church potlucks or women's retreats. I noticed if I wasn't emotionally in a place where I could enjoy my "treat" fully, I was led to abstain. But in times of celebration, surrounded by those I loved, I was led to enjoy them fully.

My emotional connection was no longer about the food, but the relationships that surrounded me.

In what used to be a place of contention and frustration, I was led to stop restricting. Because my life has nothing to do with me, this opened conversations for me and my daughters about food and the changes He was doing in me.

Eating in disciplined freedom, partnered with the Holy Spirit, became my new normal. It can be normal for you too.

- When has restriction led you into unbalanced eating?
- What would "normal eating" look like in your life? Get as detailed as possible.
- How can you invite the Holy Spirit into your food choices?
- How is God leading you into more freedom, while remaining kind to yourself?
- What would "disciplined freedom" look like in your daily life?

"For everything created by God is good, and nothing is to be rejected if it is received with gratitude"

1 Timothy 4:4

5

CREATE YOUR FOOD BOUNDARIES AND DECLARATIONS

We No Longer Live According to Rules and Restriction

AS BELIEVERS, WE GET TO LIVE in the "instead." As Isaiah 61 declares, not only did Christ liberate us from our captors and free us from our prisons, we get heaps more goodness on top of all that He did.

We get to live in the "instead."

*"Giving them a garland instead of
ashes, The oil of gladness instead
of mourning, The mantle of praise
instead of a spirit of fainting.
Instead of your shame, you will
have a double portion, And instead
of humiliation they will shout for
joy over their portion."*

Isaiah 61:3, 7

We get to take off that old self and old patterns and cycles of how we did things before and walk in the newness of life, renewed in our mind, fully knowing who we are and Whose we are. I'm sure there are times and spaces in your life where the verse in Genesis 50:20 rang true: "What Satan meant for evil, God used for good."

Reflect on other parts of your life where things were going one way, but God turned them and now you get to live in them instead.

Freedom instead of imprisonment.

A joyful and grateful heart instead of fearfully worried.

Self-control instead of being tossed to-and-fro.

Values and purpose instead of just focusing on weight loss.

What "instead" is God calling you to step into?

CREATE BOUNDARIES AND RHYTHMS FOR YOUR EMOTIONAL HEALTH

I first heard the word "boundaries" when I was in my mid-thirties. Before I learned what they are, and how to implement boundaries into my life, I lived according to whatever happened to me in life. I allowed other people's opinions, words, thoughts, and actions to determine how I viewed myself. I also went along with every thought and feeling I had, believing I had no control over them.

A few notes about boundaries:

- Your boundaries are for you, not the person next to you
- They are there to keep you and help you feel safe
- Boundaries are not walls, but a fence with a gate
- Creating and maintaining boundaries is necessary for a healthy life
- Healthy boundaries are developed in conjunction with a person's values, not fear
- Having healthy boundaries is not a one and done, but a lifestyle

To create a boundary in your life about relationships, work, health, and food you need three critical things:

- **Define your values.** You did this work in Chapter 3.
- **Assert your boundaries**. This is how you communicate your boundaries: written, verbal, or non-verbal; firm and protective, yet flexible and receptive.
- **Honor your boundaries.** Consistent decisions to maintain your values and boundaries no matter the circumstance of life.

In this chapter, we will take what we have learned so far and create boundaries for yourself and around your eating habits. These are not hard-lined rules or more promises for you to break with yourself. Think of boundaries as rhythms that you want to start walking with, to keep you healthy and moving towards victory over food, dieting, and emotional eating.

Your boundary is a line in the sand: what you will and will not do or allow.

Your rhythm is the pattern or action you will take to consistently walk out your boundary.

Because we are working on taking off the old self, being renewed in the spirit of our minds, and putting on the new self, you will identify your old patterns and the "instead" that you will begin to walk in.

It is helpful to look at your old pattern of coping and implement its replacement in a sentence. You are beginning to teach your brain a new way of doing and thinking; identifying the replacement action will help you navigate to your renewed pattern quicker. By attaching your will, you are notifying yourself on all levels, "This is the way we are going now."

Create your emotional care boundary:

Based on your Why and values, what is a boundary you need/want to put into place to keep you emotionally healthy and not using food?

Instead of ________________, I will ________________.

(e.g., Instead of using food to numb my anxiety, I will take a time out. Instead of eating my feelings after a hard day, I will relax healthily.)

Create your rhythm (the action of walking it out)

Based on your Why, values and your emotional boundary, what is/are the action step(s) you will take? Be as detailed and specific as possible.

Instead of ____________, I will ____________ by:

-
-
-

(e.g., Instead of using food to numb my anxiety, I will take a time out by:

- Removing myself from the kitchen completely
- Going for a walk, listening to worship music, or having quiet time in my room
- Checking in with a friend)

(e.g., Instead of eating my feelings after a hard day, I will relax healthily by:

- Journaling my feelings and praying through them
- Taking a bath, calling a friend, or reading a book
- Taking a walk with the dog, or going to a fitness class)

You are proactively creating an emotional boundary, a plan of action, and options to hold your boundary in place.

"The Lord is the portion of my inheritance and my cup; You support my lot. The lines have fallen to me in pleasant places; Indeed, my heritage is beautiful to me."

Psalm 16:5-6

CREATE YOUR FOOD BOUNDARIES

Based on your newfound awareness of your emotional eating patterns, you will prayerfully create food boundaries. This is not something you may be able to fully grasp and implement right away. Please understand that as we practice these principles, you will gain more ground toward victory. None of these practices should involve perfectionism, or pride that we do this on our own. The longer I walk out my journey, the more I find I need God and His strength and grace.

With your emotional plan in place, you can begin to create your food boundaries. Since emotional eating has little to do with food and much to do with feelings, we separate our boundaries for crucial self-care.

By now, you have learned the difference between your hungers and what you need to satisfy each. You also dare to lay down what does not truly satisfy. You have recognized core fears, and reasons why you eat, and hopefully all shame has been removed.

Paying attention to your health will be a lifelong process. As we heal emotionally, we often become aware of a need to heal physically. As we age, our bodies require less of some things, and more of others. We will find ourselves moving towards balance and holistic health, rather than just a certain waistline.

When we create food boundaries, we are not turning to diet-culture nonsense that our old self likes to fall into. We will gather up our true nature, who and Whose we are, our Kingdom-focused Why and values, to declare how we will fuel our bodies.

Don't fall for the trap that food boundaries need to be restrictive—they need to be life-giving. If your food boundaries are overly restrictive, if they are killing, stealing, robbing some joy and life from you, I ask you to take those to the Lord and see what He says. You may have one food boundary that keeps you safe from falling into over-eating, or you may have five boundaries. I suggest you begin with one, learning the mechanics of the one boundary and consistently abiding by it.

Here are a few questions to help you create your food boundary:

- Based on your patterns, what time of day do your struggle the most with emotional eating?
- What are your trigger emotions, and what do they lead you to consume?
- What are your trigger foods that if you had one bite, would lead you into a binge?
- Is there a certain restaurant or food that tempts you into a full-out binge?
- When I feel _________ I eat __________.

Ok, you've recognized some more patterns. Let's flip the tables and bring the Holy Spirit in.

Prayerfully ask:

- Lord, what does my body need for health and godliness?
- Lord, what boundary do I need to put in place to fuel my body?
- What is the best boundary I can put into place for my victory?
- How can I steward my body well, for the calling you have placed on my life?

Or the simple and to the point:

- Holy Spirit what is my food boundary?

Your boundary should be as simple, concise, and direct as you can make it. Remember, you are drawing a line in standing up for yourself and your health, not falling into restriction or fear. **Your boundary is a solution to a pattern that does not lead you towards health and life.**

Here are a few examples that the Holy Spirit led my clients to establish for their food boundaries:

Have you identified a time of day when emotional eating/binging is at its highest? Consider a time boundary:

- *I eat three meals per day and stop eating when satisfied.*
- *I eat according to my meal plan.*
- *I eat according to the Hunger Scale; I start eating at a 1 and stop eating at a 4.*

Maybe you identified that eating a certain food will trigger you into a binge or over-consuming:

- *I only consume refined sugar on Friday afternoons, and I have one serving.*
- *The only eat sweet foods I consume have natural sugars, such as fruit.*
- *I portion packaged foods, rather than eating out of boxes or bags.*

Do you need a boundary in place for health reasons?

- *I pack my lunch every day, rather than going to a restaurant.*
- *I fill half my plate with vegetables.*
- *I eat gluten-free.*

CREATE YOUR FOOD DECLARATIONS

I have been around the block enough times to know that staying at the surface, in the shallows, will get you nowhere fast. To create deep and lasting change, we must pull up roots of our beliefs and their offshoots. We have to replenish the soil, bring some air and water in before we can plant a seed and expect it to grow.

The work you have been doing is hard labor. You've found things growing that you don't want to be there and have dug down to pull up the root and its offshoots. We've been cultivating knowledge, truth, and new perspectives. In faith, your boundary is like a seed that you've planted.

We want to give your seed every opportunity to root, sprout, and grow into something that will bear fruit and multiply.

In John 15:4, Jesus said, "Abide in Me, and I in you. As the branch cannot bear fruit of itself unless it abides in the vine, so neither can you unless you abide in Me."

To water your seed and allow it to fully root, we need to anchor your boundary to who you are—not just what you will or will not do.

Being a man or woman who is free from emotional eating and has victory over food is an identity; it is already who you are. You can identify yourself as free, victor, and overcomer. For your brain and belief system to slide over to this realization, your behavior must match. As you gain more ground and prove to yourself your new nature, it will become easier to believe, "This is who I am, and this is what I do around food."

Do you no longer identify yourself as someone that emotionally eats?

Has the narrative around yourself and food been updated?

Ask the Holy Spirit what He says about who you are.

~

To imprint and root down your new nature, you will make declarations. They may feel not true at first, but by reciting them, practicing what you preach, and doing it consistently, you will see change on a holistic level. What you think, how you talk, what you believe, and how you act will change.

Pull out your papers with your Why, values, and boundaries.

Declare who you are. Declare what you do (and maybe do

not do). Declare the habits the real you, the true you, the victor, have with food.

For example: "I am a God-fearing woman who takes care of herself on all levels. I want to live my life energetically and fully for all my days, running into Heaven, not shuffling. I am a woman who has dedicated her life to helping and serving those in her community and I will steward what is my responsibility in health, wholeness, and wellness, surrendering all of myself back to the Lord. I am a woman who values my relationship with God, my husband, and my children. I also value honesty, integrity, and hard work. I am a woman who takes care of herself emotionally; honoring not stuffing how I feel. I am a woman who eats when I am hungry, stops when I am satisfied. I choose food that is whole and nutrient-dense, but also lives balanced with the occasional dessert. I am a woman who takes care of her body, I move it daily, but am only focused on strength, mobility, flexibility, and cardiovascular health."

Creating your food declarations is not just about changing behavior, but recognizing the truth of who you are and removing identities and habits that belong to someone else. It is easy to identify ourselves with our behaviors and habits, but the reality is that you are not a person that has an eating disorder. You are not a person that emotionally eats, but a person that is learning how to take care of yourself in a new way. Your thoughts and behaviors are changing and updating, you are changing the trajectory of your life, one choice at a time.

By making those choices with the foundational truth of who you are, it's easier to choose better. Nothing can define us unless we let it, and it can then proceed into bondage. Because we were given free will at our creation, we can choose to stop and never go back. We can take off those old grave clothes and begin wearing our robes of righteousness, especially because that's how God sees us, in Christ.

I am hoping by now you can see yourself and your old patterns in a new light. I pray that you look at yourself with the lenses of grace, love, and truth, as your Father in Heaven does. Most cases of emotional eating are rooted in survival. Since we now choose to thrive rather than just survive, we declare how we eat based on who we are.

Your food declarations are identity-based and health-focused, remembering your emotional boundary.

- Read your Kingdom-focused Why and Why Not
- Prayerfully make a declaration about who you are
- Attach your will and your reason for why you will/will not continue certain behaviors.
- Attach a scripture or word to solidify it.

Create your food boundary, based on your declaration, beginning with who you are, and ending with why you choose this.

I am _____________, I (food boundary), because

_________________________________.

For example: "I am forgiven and free, I no longer eat in emotion, because taking care of myself is a kingdom work that I get to steward. 'Who the Son sets free is free indeed.')"

Create your declaration with as much detail as you want. You can write a paragraph or a one-liner. This will be something you recite every day, and you will also wield it during times when emotions/stress/temptation are building or are at their highest. Your declaration is a tool for your tool belt that you will use whenever necessary.

*"The LORD is the portion of my
inheritance and my cup;
You support my lot.
The measuring lines have
fallen for me in pleasant
places;
Indeed, my inheritance is
beautiful to me."*

Psalm 16:5-6

CREATE NEW RHYTHMS WITH FOOD

Emotional eating, dieting, and falling off the wagon all tell us that we can't trust ourselves. Every time we sign up for a diet, begin another "Day One," and eventually break our own promises, we trust ourselves less and less. It may even cause us to stop trusting God as our ever-present help. These "breaks," or times when we didn't do what we said we would do, creates a momentum that is bent on breaking our agreements.

Before someone becomes a client of mine, I ask, "What do you need from me?" Everyone answers in their way, but "accountability" is infused throughout their answer.

It's so much easier to be trusted when someone else is holding us accountable to our agreements. But what happens when that accountability is gone, and you are only accountable to yourself again? We have been working on this part of your food freedom since the beginning—the Lord is holding you accountable for everything he has entrusted to you.

- What have you been entrusted to steward or what you are responsible for every day, or a large part of your life? E. g., marriage, children, ministry, job, finances, pets, relationships with family members and friends, etc.

- What areas of your life can you be fully trusted to show up every day and offer your best?
- Is it different from your eating habits or food choices?
- Write down the victories you have had in your life with your food choices. These could be from five years ago, or five minutes ago.
- Your brain, and often the enemy, will only point out the failures. Shame is a natural emotion, and we can use it to change our behavior, or we can allow it to take us down and take us out.
- Why is the narrative that you cannot be trusted with food wrong?
- Tell me why you *can* be trusted with food.

Keys to taking back and rebuilding trust around food:

- Understand there is no pass or fail with eating.
- There are no good or bad foods. Food is completely neutral; it is our body's response that determines which foods are good or bad for us, individually.
- Some foods will give us a high; those foods are usually what our brains get addicted to, and they become a hard pattern to break.
- Food is a physical source of sustaining life and cannot make us feel anything emotionally.
- Focus on nutrition, not emotional stability.
- Critique, not criticize; be aware of what you are doing and why you are doing it, but don't hold yourself back and down by judging yourself harshly.

Rebuilding trust with yourself around food will take time. Often, we must listen to the narrative in our brain that wants to classify our goodness according to our habits and behaviors. That is why we made boundaries and declarations based on who we *are*, not what we *do*. Creating new rhythms around food, it is often one choice and one meal at a time, in the beginning. Asking God for His strength and help before making a food choice is wisdom. Invite the Holy Spirit into your food choices and at the table while you dine. These actions form new rhythms, new habits, and eventually a new lifestyle of trusting yourself with your choices around food and how to take care of yourself.

"For I desire mercy, not sacrifice, and acknowledgment of God rather than burnt offerings."

Hosea 6:6 NIV

6

REFRAME OLD MINDSETS

Retrain Your Body and Mind to Operate in Godly Peace

The battlefield for your freedom will always be in your mind. Whether it's the enemy of your soul poking at pain points or conditioning leading you into self-sabotage, your thoughts are what drive your life and determine where you are going.

In Psalm 56, we get a clear picture of David acknowledging his feelings, thinking his thoughts, and taking an extensive inventory of what was going on around him. He felt and knew that he was afraid, but chose to come up higher. David is a prime example of a person well-acquainted with his thoughts and feelings, taking them captive, bringing them to the Lord, and reframing them based on his faith in God.

*"When I am afraid, I will put my
trust in You. In God, whose word I
praise, in God I have put my trust; I
shall not be afraid, what can mere
man do to me?"*

Psalm 56:3-4

Our thoughts lead to feelings, which can lead to action or inaction. Our thoughts are where we defuse our feelings, and can choose to continue despite them.

We have created boundaries and set our food declarations into motion, and at some point, all of this will come under fire. We will be tempted to allow our thoughts and emotions to control us again, sending us back into emotional eating. We will feel the resistance inside our bodies—overwhelm, or anxiety—but even in those moments we have a choice. It's in those moments where our response counts the most.

SEPARATE FROM THE LIES

You have done so much work reframing how you think about yourself, your life, and your food. You have created your food plan, declaring how, when, and what you will or will not be eating. Knowing that you have a choice, you can insert yourself between the world around you, and the world within you, taking huge strides towards victory.

When we make our new and exciting plans, things can start out feeling easy and we think, "I've got this!"

But when your plan comes under fire, this is a point of temptation to go back to your old ways, or hold steady to your agreements of victory and freedom.

We do this by:

- Reading aloud our Why Statement and envisioning the life that is ours
- Proactively exposing the voice that will come to sabotage our efforts
- Writing down a series of "reasons" we won't be able to adhere to our plan
- Understanding that these lies come from the saboteur and are meant to defeat us
- Replacing the lies with solution-minded thoughts and actions consistent with our identities in Christ.

The voice of the saboteur is focused on the problems and obstacles only, never the solution. This voice is helpless, hopeless, and is also an emotional driver. It creates illusions that life is too hard, and food is the only way out. The saboteur is hell-bent on taking you down and taking you out completely. It speaks in half-truths, making you think the only way out is to choose the temptation, not seeing the options God always provides.

Reframe Exercise

- Read your Why Statement out loud
- Write your Food Declarations at the top of your page
- Number your paper 1-15 down the left column

- Read your Food Declarations out loud and listen for the voice that speaks against what you are declaring. Write down what it says. Repeat this process until you get to number 15.
- Go back through the list of lies the saboteur fed you, replacing each lie with the truth. You can explain why this is a lie, and how you won't fall for it in the future.
- Add scripture to replace the lies, solidifying with God's truth.
- Keep this page handy, referring to it each morning to proactively renew your mind and replace lies with truth.

Throughout your day, identity your thoughts asking, "Is this me, or the saboteur?" Find the lie and replace it with the truth. You can add a reframe to your declarations, making a solid rebuke and refuting whenever you need one. I have found the harsher the lie, the harsher my refute must be. This is where the tension in the separation is found. The tension is us allowing our minds to be renewed while taking off the old-self and putting on the new-self. The enemy and saboteur want nothing more than for you to stay down and stuck in bondage. This is where you rise above, this is where you use fighting words and commit overcome this battle waging within you.

You will eventually notice a theme to the saboteur since there is nothing new under the sun. Sometimes it will get sneaky. Take your time, take a breath, and practice refuting it.

To take it one step further: do this exercise every morning, but instead of fifteen, listen for 3-5 lies the saboteur is giving you, and replace them with the truth.

The enemy will always call you out, but God will always call you up.

> *"For though we walk in the flesh, we do*
> *not wage battle according to the flesh,*
> *for the weapons of our warfare are not*
> *of the flesh, but divinely powerful for the*
> *destruction of fortresses. We are*
> *destroying arguments and all arrogance*
> *raised against the knowledge of God,*
> *and we are taking every thought captive*
> *to the obedience of Christ, and we are*
> *ready to punish all disobedience,*
> *whenever your obedience is complete."*
>
> *2 Corinthians 10:3-6*

SELF-DISCIPLINE IS NOT THE "S" WORD

The word discipline has gotten a bad rap.

I used to equate discipline with punishment. Now I know they are separate, and discipline is now welcomed in my life. Discipline, if done correctly, is a teacher and allows for growth. It allows you to make mistakes while learning how to choose better next time.

I have said becoming a runner taught me self-discipline.

But in digging deeper into the thought, I *allowed* running to teach me self-discipline.

Anything in our lives can be used to teach us and grow us into more discipline, bringing fullness, multiplication, and bearing good fruit. Tapping into self-control or self-discipline allows us to show ourselves that we can do something and prove that we can continue doing it.

Our mindset shift:

I can't do this-> I am doing this-> I can do this-> I did this.

Self-discipline does not mean knowing everything you need to know and doing it perfectly. Self-discipline is showing up every day and doing what you can do, then going a little further than you did yesterday. It's all about the choice you made to show up for yourself and obey what the Lord is calling you to do. Self-discipline in *Food Freedom* comes from deciding you are no longer an emotional eater and living a life according to that decision, no matter if you feel like it or not—because food is no longer an option unless it pertains to physical hunger.

Getting to that place of freedom requires new beginnings, small steps, getting specific, and being consistent day in and day out, until it is part of who you are.

Self-discipline is a choice not based on circumstance, feelings, or impulses, but on our godly standard of living. We align ourselves with this choice, and set our sights and goals on things above. We make choices according to who we are and God's calling on our life—eternal, not temporal.

FOOD FREEDOM

*"For this reason, I remind you to kindle
afresh the gift of God which is in you
through the laying on of my hands. For
God has not given us a spirit of timidity,
but of power and love and discipline."*

2 Timothy 1:6-7

Freedom takes consistent daily effort to refute what attempts to lure you back into bondage. Don't believe the lie that there is an easy button in freedom because there isn't. Jesus died for our freedom, and now we get to flesh out this freedom with our lives. Self-discipline is often tricky to figure out until you are in it, working that muscle. But is in the testing that our discipline muscles are tried and torn to become stronger.

*"For the moment, all discipline seems not
to be pleasant, but painful; yet to those
who have been trained by it, afterward it
yields the peaceful fruit of righteousness.
Therefore, strengthen the hands that are
weak and the knees that are feeble, and
make straight paths for your feet, so that
the limb, which is impaired may not be
dislocated, but rather be healed."*
Hebrews 12:11-13

CONSISTENCY IS KEY

We have learned the mechanics of food freedom, created our food plan, healthy coping mechanisms, and set boundaries. You have learned that new beginnings don't have to be overwhelming or carry the fear of failure; they can be fun and exciting!

Learning the mechanics of something new and doing them consistently is the key to making lasting change.

Our brains like to feel safe and at rest, knowing what is coming. Our emotions like to come into a rhythmic hum of one plus one is two. All the guessing is gone, the what-ifs are put to rest, and we know that if we work our plan consistently, we will be successful.

It's when we throw intensity in the mix that things get chaotic and overwhelming. Adding intensity too soon may throw off our cumulative work and send us back to the drawing board, believing that our initial plan wasn't good enough.

When I first started working out my own food freedom, I was happy just not .

My goal was to not binge, period. And so, day in and day out, my focus and intention for the day were to do everything I could to not binge. I had my food plan, my way of escape when emotions and tensions got high, and my self-care plan with coping mechanisms in place. I had a plan that worked at home, and at the hospital when I was there with my daughter. I had a plan that worked when we went out to restaurants and when I sat down to a holiday meal. I had my mechanics down pat, and my will was set on remaining consistent, checking that box every day and night.

After a while, I felt a nudge to attempt to try to lose weight. This nudge wasn't from the Holy Spirit, but just myself dipping my toe into waters, seeing if I could manage the temperature of the weight loss pool.

My focus moved from "just don't binge," to "just don't binge and try to lose weight."

I was unable to do it at first. Working on losing weight was too much for me to handle at the time, along with the rest of what I was juggling. But out of those "failures," came my recovery plan—a plan of action for how I would pick myself back up after a binge. Because the biggest problem with is not one mistake or mishap. It's not one meal, or even one day of eating. The issue is if we consistently live in self-harm rather than self-discipline. We can live in freedom even if our freedom is walked out 50% of the time. Because each time you pick yourself back up, you are learning how to recover better and faster. You will eventually go from 50% to 55%, 60%, 65%, and so forth. You will not be living in bondage anymore, but slowly and consistently breaking free. You may visit emotional eating from time to time. That's okay, because you don't live there anymore.

You don't have to worry that you failed or fell off some invisible wagon—if you learned something, it was a lesson. Not only are you working your self-discipline muscle, but you are also building your resilience.

- Start with small achievable tasks, like your food boundaries and declarations, and do them consistently for an extended period of time. Start with thirty days and work your way up to fully changing your lifestyle.
- Adopt the mindset that you are learning something new and retraining your brain. Some days will be harder than others, but after a while, you will have adopted these practices as your own.
- Make changes prayerfully; you will always need the strength of the Lord to get you through.

Only once you've practiced your new habit consistently for at least 30 days should you add any intensity or change things up. Self-disciplined people have a plan, work it consistently, and it becomes who they are. Success is never an accident. Working your *Food Freedom* plan every day and picking yourself right back up when you need to are crucial.

SIT IN THE RESISTANCE

As former emotional eaters, our brains were hard-wired into fight or flight—feel the emotion, fly to food, repeat.

It is hard work to de-escalate our emotions with our rational thinking, feel the resistance in our bodies, and not take the path to food for comfort.

When making this change, it can feel like we are going against everything we know what to do to take care of ourselves. We can lash out unexpectedly, have anxiety, and feel panic. When we stop turning to food in our emotions and choose to feel them and process through them, our old ways come against us. But this is where we remain strong. You are rewiring your brain and the way that it deals and copes with emotion. You are rewiring neural pathways that have been your coping superhighway for however long you've been pacifying yourself this way. It is incredibly uncomfortable, but the good news is that you are not alone and you are doing amazing work.

After years of working to get free, the Holy Spirit revealed to me that I was using food to cover up an extreme anxiety disorder. When I decided to no longer use food to numb my feelings, guess what was waiting for me: extreme anxiety. Since I knew better than to continue to use food, I had to choose differently and take care of myself emotionally.

Being a person that found comfort in chaos, I could scapegoat my anxiety on what was going on around me, rather than what was going on internally. I even created anxiety when there was none to be found because rest was foreign to me. Rest was scary because rest reveals the truth. Rest revealed yokes I'd inadvertently taken upon myself and was attached to. Rest revealed the weight I was carrying and how heavy the load had been.

The antidote to my anxiety was to do nothing, just sit still and breathe.

"Feel it, Lindsay, feel all of this and do nothing about it," the Holy Spirit whispered. "I've got you, I'm with you in this, don't be afraid."

Sitting still with a brain on fire, a body shaking, while forcing my breath to go deeper into my lungs was the beginning. I knew I was healing something in my brain, retraining my habits, and that only good could come out of the work.

I call this sitting in the resistance or wait-lifting (yes, I spelled that right).

Sitting in the resistance is a practice you have been learning throughout your journey in *Food Freedom*. You have sat with hard feelings, processed through emotions, and made decisions not to eat despite wanting to. You have emotionally picked up heavy things, sat under the weight of them, put them down, and picked up another heavy thing. The stuff you walk through every day is heavy, and you have been choosing the hard and narrow path to lift these things, rather than run from them.

Sitting in the resistance is continuing to do the work when you don't feel like it. Sometimes we do it for the sake of consistency, but most of the time it's to practice living according to who we truly are within a life we want to live.

> *"For the moment, all discipline seems not to be pleasant, but painful; yet to those who have been trained by it, afterward it yields the peaceful fruit of righteousness."*
>
> *Hebrews 12:11*

To think these new ways of living won't come under fire is simply not wise. Our brains don't like to do new things or uncomfortable things, but for a time they will come along with us. We have been making small adjustments, lifting one- or two-pound weights repeatedly. But life has a way of happening, and these new habits will come under fire and will be tested. It's like our brains are ready to click over, but are making one last attempt, saying, "Are you sure this is what we are doing now? Because what we were doing before was more comfortable and I was used to it." It is at this point, where we sit in the resistance and choose to push through, rather than back down and head into food bondage again.

Hebrews 12:7 tell us "It is for discipline that you endure."

By sitting in the resistance, we are building endurance so that we may become disciplined.

This is the testing and training part of our journey that we move through to get to the other side. Each time we go after more healing, more freedom, or more joy, what we used to know and how we used to operate will come under fire and be put to the test.

Not only do we test our own will, but the enemy does too.

~

God does not tempt us to sin. That would go against His holy nature and contrary to His desire for us to be holy as He is. The goal of our Christian walk is to not fall into temptation but follow God into His way of doing, being, and living. He can certainly allow the enemy to lead us into temptation and test our will and desire to choose Him instead.

Jesus was led into the wilderness to be tempted and tested for 40 days and nights. What makes us think our wills won't be tested? The disciples asked Jesus how they should pray. Jesus responded, "and lead us not into temptation but deliver us from evil." This part of the prayer reveals the petition of the believer to avoid sin altogether. It also implies that God has control over the tempter and saves us when we call upon Him.

> *"No temptation has overtaken you*
> *except something common to mankind;*
> *and God is faithful, so He will not allow*
> *you to be tempted beyond what you are*
> *able, but with the temptation will*
> *provide the way of escape also, so that*
> *you will be able to endure it."*
>
> *1 Corinthians 10:13*

Temptation can also be referred to as trials. We know that God will not test us beyond our ability to withstand, and along with the temptation we also get a way out.

When I read this scripture, I picture both of my hands outstretched, palms facing up. In my left hand, temptation and all that goes along with it: thoughts, feelings, emotions, and shame. The temptation is often easier to choose and feels good to the flesh. In my right hand is God's way out of the temptation. This choice feels harder to accept in my flesh, and the reach for it is longer and more drawn out than the temptation.

It would be so much easier if you could see the fruit of each of these choices, but once you make the choice fruition will come. You either passed the test and didn't take the temptation, or you learned more about the bait for next time. Temptation is a test and God gets the glory each time His kids choose Him, rather than the enemy's bait.

> *"But to those who rebuke the wicked will be delight, and a good blessing will come upon them."*
>
> *Proverbs 24:25*
>
> *"Submit therefore to God. Resist the devil, and he will flee from you."*
>
> *James 4:7*

Whenever we pray, believe, or go after more in the Kingdom of God, and freedom in Christ, it will come under fire and will be tested. We can laugh through some testing times, while other days it can feel like you were hit by a garbage truck. I have often been on the other side of extreme resistance, finally able to see that the attack was just a test of my will and resolve to follow God and the word He spoke to me.

- Prayerfully ask the Lord what scripture or word you are to hold onto in your time of testing and need.
- Prayerfully ask the Lord for His way out when resistance comes. Ask Him for a plan, an idea of what to do in the heat of the moment.
- How can you reframe your thinking now, proactively, before the testing and resistance come?
- What is the course of action you will take when resistance comes for your food freedom? Write down what you will do and resolve to save it to memory.

"But seek first His kingdom and His righteousness, and all these things will be provided to you."

Matthew 6:33

Heavenly Father, Your Word says that you will always provide for us a way out when we are tempted. Please make your way known to us and help us choose and submit to You, and You alone. Your word says that when we submit to you, the enemy will flee from us, so Lord we release our will to choose You every single time. Grant us greater discernment, and help us sit in the resistance that comes against us. May we grow stronger and more able to withstand more, so that we may bring you glory with our lives and with our choices day in and day out. In Jesus Name, Amen.

7

CREATE YOUR RECOVERY PLAN

Your Healing is in Your Going

Humanity.

Our humanity required a recovery and rescue mission. God had a plan and He executed it perfectly. You and I have a plan, and because of our humanity, we will not. It's okay, grace upon grace.

A recovery plan is helpful to add to your existing plan. It is a fail-safe: not that you won't fall, but that you will pick yourself back up in a dramatic fashion in the next meal or the next day. You might get down, but you won't stay down.

The world likes to throw out more restrictions to "fix" the calories of a binge. It can offer you fasting, long workouts, starvation and creating plans out of fear. But we don't do that anymore.

Your recovery day should follow your boundaries and declarations, only readjusting if a trigger needs to be addressed. The best thing you can do for yourself, in recovering from a binge, to move you towards healing, is eat rather than starving yourself to "fix" the binge. Remember you're doing a lot of work to feel your feelings without eating, create new habits, and still maintain your day-to-day life.

True recovery is done in kindness and compassion.

It can look like:

- Drinking more water to help your body process through the extra food
- Going for a gentle walk to boost your mood
- Taking a nap or resting if fatigued
- Acknowledging your feelings and processing through

Adding restriction or quick fixes to your recovery plan, or making this about your body, could lead you into another binge.

You are in recovery for a reason, something must have happened to send you here. By taking care of yourself in a compassionate way, you will be able to rebound quickly and not carry emotional eating into the next day.

Healing is an ongoing rhythm. One day you feel happy and free, the next you are crying on the kitchen floor—allow room for both.

Gaining and maintaining health is an ongoing rhythm. There is always be room for recalculations to help us get better and feel better. Don't be afraid to try new things. Be a beginner at something, learn a new way of doing things—it can open you up to so many possibilities. Be in a rhythm of prayerfully growing and learning. Remain a student of life because the Teacher will always appear when the student is ready.

Have fun with the process. Not only are you learning so much more about yourself, you are allowing God into spaces of your life that He will use. Allow yourself the time to learn what you need to learn, so that you can fully take back your territory of freedom, stewarding your health and total well-being.

Remain kind to yourself.

Remain rooted in Christ.

Remain intimate with Him.

Remain in your identity in Christ, who you are, not what you do or what you look like.

Remain free from bondage, don't get sucked into fruitless things.

"You are already clean because of the word which I have spoken to you. Remain in Me, and I in you. Just as the branch cannot bear fruit of itself but must remain in the vine, so neither can you unless you remain in Me. I am the vine, you are the branches; the one who remains in Me, and I in him bears much fruit, for apart from Me you can do nothing." John 15:3-5

I believe in you. Do you believe in you?

Abide in freedom and victory because they are yours.

Peace be with you always!

ABOUT THE AUTHOR

Lindsay Wendland lives in Somerset, WI with her husband, Nathan, and their three daughters. They also share their home with two dogs and a cat who thinks he's a dog. Lindsay enjoys the outdoors in their fullest capacity by running, hiking, biking, and gardening.

As a Master Coach in Holistic Health, Lindsay has devoted herself for over a decade to taking back her territory from emotional eating and the havoc it creates in the body. She has developed a coaching program specifically designed to help those get free and stay free from all emotional eating.
For self-paced, group, or one on one coaching head over to takebackyourterritory.com/coaching

To listen to Lindsay's teachings on Food Freedom, find Biblical inspiration, and to go further in your freedom journey check out the Take Back Your Territory Podcast wherever you stream your favorite shows!